HEALING
MASSAGE

HEALING MASSAGE

Simple Techniques to Soothe Pain
and Find Relief at Home

JENNIFER LOVE, CMT, NMT, NMTHE

Illustrations by Christy Ni

ROCKRIDGE
PRESS

For general information on our other products and services or to obtain technical support, please contact our Customer Care Department within the United States at (866) 744-2665, or outside the United States at (510) 253-0500.

Rockridge Press publishes its books in a variety of electronic and print formats. Some content that appears in print may not be available in electronic books, and vice versa.

TRADEMARKS: Rockridge Press and the Rockridge Press logo are trademarks or registered trademarks of Callisto Media Inc. and/or its affiliates, in the United States and other countries, and may not be used without written permission. All other trademarks are the property of their respective owners. Rockridge Press is not associated with any product or vendor mentioned in this book.

Interior and Cover Designer: Peatra Jariya
Art Producer: Megan Baggott
Editor: Rachel Feldman
Production Editor: Rachel Taenzler

Illustration © 2020 Christy Ni
Author photo courtesy of Caitlyn Tweedy

ISBN: Print 978-1-64611-188-6 | eBook 978-1-64611-189-3

R0

—

To the glory of God,
who brought me back to life.

To the love of my life, Calith,
who lights me up.

To the women who show me how to
Believe, Belong, and Become.

And to my children,
Jefferson, Jackson, and Joshua, who teach me daily
that my life's true purpose is love, motherhood,
snuggling, and nailing it.

—

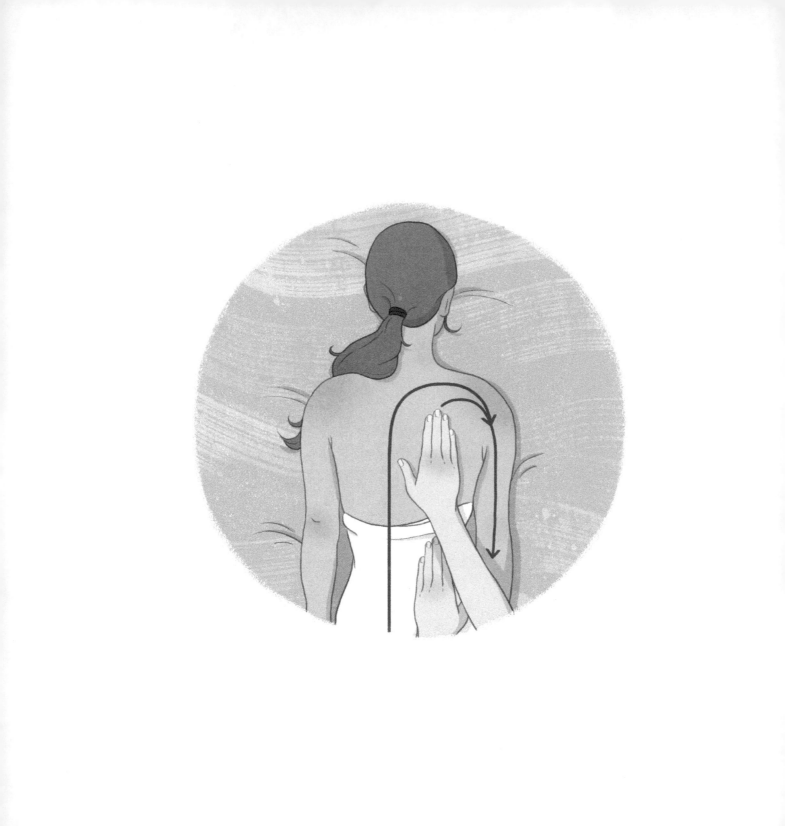

Contents

Introduction

Perhaps you have come to this book in chronic pain, searching for an alternative therapy because so many pills and scans haven't made a difference. Maybe you deal with a disorder and are looking for ways to find relief from its symptoms. Or perhaps you're looking for a new coping skill to deal with stress, anxiety, or another aspect of mental health.

I'm here to tell you that massage is a powerful tool for healing. This book will help you harness that tool with tips, tricks, and techniques for performing massage at home on yourself or on a loved one who needs relief.

In addition to teaching at a premier massage therapy college in California, I run a medical massage therapy clinic in midtown Sacramento. Massage changed my life, too. I took a (stress)full load of advanced high school classes and tests, headed off to an expensive four-year college to get a bachelor's degree, then launched myself directly into an expensive law school, expecting to spend my life in a small office producing documents and paying off student loans until I expired.

As the years passed in my law practice, our culture of chronic stress took its toll on me, particularly when combined with my childhood trauma and a crushing amount of student loan debt. I spent my early adult life dealing with frequent bouts of depression, anxiety, and suicidal thoughts. After 14 years of high-octane performance, I decided I no longer wanted to run in the rat race; chronic pain, irritable bowel syndrome (exacerbated by extreme stress), carpal tunnel syndrome, thoracic outlet syndrome, and full-body muscle aches and pains sent me frequently to the emergency room and interfered with my work, relationships, and parenting.

After nearly three decades in the fight-flight-or-freeze zone, I learned what it meant to rest. I became a yoga teacher and yoga therapist, specializing in restorative yoga to heal people with stillness. I found peace in my faith. I spent years in talk therapy, unraveling the negative thoughts and unhealthy habits I had developed while operating in survival mode. I came to massage therapy school in the middle of that process, ready to learn some extra tools for my yoga tool belt. When my own physical and emotional ailments eased through daily massage, I found a calling. I realized that my career's purpose lay in being the healing hands and feet that help people get in touch with the best version of themselves through massage therapy and health education.

When I graduated from the advanced neuromuscular therapy program at my college with 1,350 hours of massage training, I opened my own medical massage clinic. I now work with doctors, chiropractors, physical therapists, and other health-care professionals to educate them and their patients on the benefits and healing power of massage. People come to my clinic because they know they will be listened to, supported, and guided well on their path to optimum health and wellness.

This book is for anyone looking for healing massage techniques to use at home, but it is written specifically for you: someone with little to no experience in massage. I've included basic introductory information to get you started, easy-to-understand instructions with illustrations for every technique, self-care tips for each ailment, and information on great extras like essential oils and hot stones.

I believe you or your loved one will find unexpected relief at home in no time using this book.

Thank you for trusting me to be a part of your healing journey—it is a responsibility I do not take lightly. It is my heartfelt prayer that you will pass your knowledge and massage on to those around you, continuing to spread the healing power of touch in a world that desperately needs to rediscover it.

Please note that the recommendations in this book are not intended to cure any disease or replace your current medications. Always consult with your doctor before embarking on a new healing protocol.

PART 1

The Power of Touch

Welcome to the next step on your journey to healing. Massage is a powerful tool that has been used for centuries to soothe and relieve painful ailments from anxiety and stress to injuries and chronic pain. In part 1 of this book, I will prepare you mentally and physically to give a massage, so you will be able to apply the specific massage techniques and tips in part 2.

Chapter 1 introduces you to popular and effective styles of massage throughout the ages and helps you understand how to use massage for healing at home, including tips for addressing chronic pain.

Chapter 2 covers basic anatomy, including what creates a "knot" in your muscles, and important techniques you can use right now to relieve pain and relax your partner

during massage. It includes special considerations for massaging yourself, as well as pregnant, elderly, or young partners.

Chapter 3 helps you prepare yourself and your environment to give a safe, comfortable, and effective massage. It also discusses extras you can use to enhance your massage, including essential oils and hot and cold therapy.

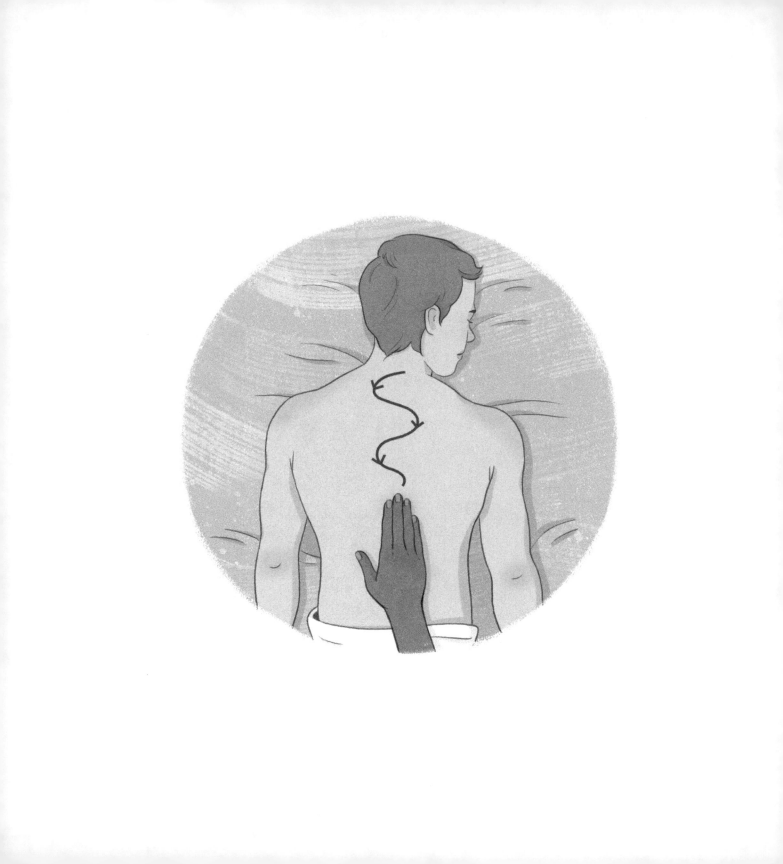

CHAPTER 1

Massage for Healing

Welcome to the next step on your journey to healing. Massage is a powerful tool that has been used for centuries to soothe and relieve painful ailments, from anxiety and stress to injuries and chronic pain. This chapter will introduce you to the world of massage, including its history, its many styles, and how it is used around the world today.

WHAT IS MASSAGE?

Massage is touch therapy, i.e., the use of touch to manipulate the soft tissues of the body, stimulate the relaxation response of the nervous system, and restore balance to the body and mind. Throughout human history, massage has been used in Eastern and Western cultures to relieve emotional, mental, and physical suffering. From ancient Egyptian pictographs showing hand and foot massage to Chinese athletes wearing purple spots from cupping therapy at modern-day Olympic games, we see people turning to massage to care for their bodies.

For the past few decades, massage has been treated as **complementary and alternative medicine** (CAM) because health-care professionals falsely have believed the lack of scientific research means massage is unlikely to benefit their patients. Doctors and chiropractors have sent their patients to massage therapists as a last resort, after years of pain, pills, scans, and surgeries that were unable to heal their pain.

This situation was created in part because as the medical field developed, there was no doctor of skeletal muscles. Every major system of the body (there are 11) except **muscles** has its own specialty, like neurology (nerves), orthopedics (bones), and cardiology (heart muscle). Muscles were treated lightly in medical school, and quickly forgotten as doctors trained and practiced in their specialty.

Today, massage is increasingly used in **integrative** health-care clinics at leading medical institutions, as scientific research on the benefits of massage has exploded over the last decade. Now health-care professionals are more educated about the benefits of massage and are more likely to refer people with acute and chronic pain to a massage therapist as a first line of defense. Research has already shown that massage may help relieve symptoms related to:

- Anxiety
- Breast cancer
- Colon and rectal surgeries
- Digestive disorders
- Fibromyalgia
- Headaches
- Heart surgery
- Insomnia related to stress
- Lower-back pain (acute and chronic)
- Myofascial pain syndrome
- Neck and shoulder pain
- Osteoarthritis of the knee
- Soft-tissue strains or injuries
- Sports injuries
- Temporomandibular joint (TMJ) pain

By reading this book, you are helping to change our society's approach to massage in health care. As an advocate for yourself and your partner, you can share with your health-care team how massage works and how it has helped you and your partner.

MASSAGE FOR HEALING

Massage therapy doesn't just feel good; it's good for you. While most people think of massage as a luxury, its reputation is changing as research proves massage has a wide range of health benefits. Most people use massage today to deal with the physical and emotional effects of our culture of chronic stress. Studies have shown that even one massage session can help heal physical and emotional ailments, from decreasing chronic pain and lowering blood pressure to reducing stress, anxiety, and depression.

Physical Health

Massage science is simple: Massage increases circulation during and immediately after the massage, which allows more nutrients and oxygen to reach the muscles and improve **lymphatic** flow (the body's plumbing and filtration system). By increasing blood flow to the muscles, knotted muscles release, which increases your strength and range of motion and reduces your pain and tension in the area. Increased blood flow also strengthens your blood vessels, which leads to lower blood pressure over time. Improved lymphatic flow reduces swelling and enhances the body's natural immune system response, helping you fight off infection and stay healthy.

CHRONIC PAIN

Often people who seek out the healing benefits of massage suffer from chronic pain. According to the Centers for Disease Control (CDC), an estimated 50 million Americans (20.4 percent of the United States's adult population) reported suffering from chronic pain in 2018. In fact, the CDC estimated that chronic pain management costs us around $560 billion each year in direct medical costs, lost productivity, and disability programs. So you are not alone in your search for an explanation and relief for your pain.

It is likely that your doctors have been unable to find the source of your pain, whether it started as a traumatic injury or came on gradually. As we touched on before, doctors do not yet specialize in muscles. It is not scientifically possible to diagnose muscle pain, tension, or trigger points using any medical scan or test. Nerve impingement as

Contraindications

Our first priority in massage is always safety, for you and your partner. Just as there are many reasons to receive a massage, there are several situations in which massage cannot be performed (**absolute contraindications** to massage). These situations include, but are not limited to, people dealing with:

- Acute pneumonia, lung abscess, or lung tumor
- Contagious, airborne, infectious disease (including flus, colds, strep throat, shingles, etc.)
- Endocarditis, pericarditis, or severe atherosclerosis
- Fever above 100.4 degrees Fahrenheit
- Hemorrhage, sepsis, or bacteremia
- Highly metastatic cancers (lymphoma, malignant melanoma, etc.)
- Infectious skin conditions (including impetigo and staph infections)
- Intoxication (drugs and alcohol)
- Meningitis or chronic active hepatitis
- Pitting edema (skin remains indented when pressed)
- Preeclampsia or eclampsia during pregnancy
- Radiation therapy (no massage during or for several weeks after treatment)
- Recent stroke, aneurysm, or heart attack
- Respiratory, liver, kidney, or other organ failure
- Severe unexplained internal pain

There are also situations where massage may be helpful, but the treatment must be modified in some way to accommodate certain health conditions (**relative contraindications** for massage), including recent injury, **bruising, or fracture**, as well as:

- **Arthritis** or osteoporosis
- Asthma, emphysema, or congestive heart failure
- Cancer
- Diabetes

- Drug withdrawal
- Epilepsy or seizure disorders
- Fibromyalgia
- High blood pressure (not controlled by medication)
- Immune system conditions
- Joint dislocation, hypermobility, or instability
- Lupus (during a flare-up)
- Lymphedema
- Neurological conditions (including decreased sensation, Bell's palsy, Parkinson's, cerebral palsy, multiple sclerosis, and spinal cord injuries)
- Pregnancy
- Raynaud's disease
- Thrombosis or phlebitis
- Use of pain medication (use lighter pressure)

Finally, sometimes massage is appropriate on most areas of the body, but a certain area must be avoided (**absolute local contraindications** for massage) due to:

- Acute inflammation
- Burns
- Deep-vein thrombosis or severe varicose veins (massage only above the site to avoid moving blood clots)
- Injuries (acute/recent)
- Lumps, cysts, or moles not diagnosed by a doctor
- Open wounds or scars
- Venomous bites or stings

If you have any doubt about whether massage is okay, hold off and consult a doctor to get the green light before massaging yourself or your partner. It's always better to be safe than sorry!

measured by electrical impulses is the closest we can get, and it is inconclusive. So for now, massage (in its many forms) is the only way to find and release this tension and thus relieve that kind of pain.

The other missing source is your brain. Our perception of pain has a complicated relationship with the nervous system. When our nerves receive a signal, they send it to the brain via the spinal cord. When the brain receives the signal, it uses many environmental and chemical factors to interpret the signal. The nerves do not send "pain signals"; the brain decides what is painful or not, and may interpret the signal as pain, itch, nausea, tickling, or even fatigue, depending on the brain's sensation of danger. Traumatic issues from your past also contribute to whether the brain interprets a signal as dangerous.

For people in chronic pain, the nervous system (brain + spinal cord + nerves) has "learned" over months and years to interpret signals as pain, even when there may not be any actual tissue damage. And to complicate things further, when signals from a certain nerve are received repeatedly, the brain may choose to send back information telling the nerve to be less sensitive, causing the pain to come and go in areas where you are accustomed to feeling pain.

For example, during times of high stress or anxiety, the brain may have less time to diminish the signals, so the pain may increase. Or the stress and anxiety may overwhelm the brain, causing the signals to end up on the back burner, resulting in decreased pain. When the pain comes and goes, it confuses you *and* your doctors!

So, yes: Your pain is real, and it is complicated. It exists in your body and mind. When your brain says, "This hurts," it does hurt, because your brain decides what you feel.

How can you change it? It's not an easy process. Using massage to eliminate sources of physical pain may help. As physical pain is released, areas of the body holding onto trauma may also let go, leading to an emotional release. You might also try **cognitive behavioral therapy** (CBT) to convince your brain you are not in danger (including changing beliefs created by traumatic situations from your past). This comprehensive approach is supported by scientific research. A study published in the *European Journal of Pain* in 2013 on **cognitive functional therapy** (CFT) for moderate back pain stated that "disabling back pain can change for the better with a different narrative and coping strategies." In fact, it said CFT was more effective than massage and exercise for "reducing pain, disability, fear beliefs, mood, and sick leave."

So there is hope. Work with your health-care team to create a new narrative, build coping skills, and include new pain treatments like massage and psychotherapy for physical, mental, and emotional health. With treatment, time, and practice, you can heal from chronic pain and be whole again.

Mental Health

Massage influences the production of several hormones. Hormones are your body's way of changing its internal environment, which changes how you feel physically and emotionally. Massage elevates levels of **dopamine**, **serotonin**, **endorphins**, and **oxytocin**. Higher levels of these hormones lead to better focus (dopamine), improved sleep, less irritability, and fewer cravings (serotonin), pain reduction and more joyful feelings (endorphins), and improved emotional stability in relationships (oxytocin).

Massage also reduces levels of **cortisol**, which is the hormone released in response to high levels of stress. In potentially dangerous situations, cortisol raises your heart rate and shuts down less essential systems like digestion, which is important in the body's fight-flight-or-freeze response. In our culture of chronic stress, this response may stay on indefinitely, putting your physical and emotional health at risk. Prolonged high levels of cortisol cause weight gain and high blood pressure, disrupt your sleep, and increase your risk of heart disease, obesity, anxiety, and depression. By reducing cortisol levels, massage protects your physical and mental health and helps heal the effects of chronic stress.

Massage Styles around the World

ACUPRESSURE, TUI NA, AND SHIATSU

Traditional Chinese Medicine holds that the body's energy, or **qi**, flows along established meridians, and dysfunction occurs when qi is stagnant or overabundant. **Acupressure** at specific points on the meridians was developed to move qi, bring the body and mind into balance, and address specific conditions that arise from this *dis*-ease. Acupressure is typically done on a floor mat with the recipient clothed. Chinese **tui na** uses rhythmic compressions and acupressure to massage soft tissue and improve energy flow. Japanese **shiatsu** uses finger pressure to move the body's energy along meridians to restore balance and health.

AYURVEDIC MASSAGE

Ayurveda is an ancient system of medicine in India that prescribes daily and seasonal regimens depending on a person's constitution. Massage is an important aspect of Ayurvedic medicine. It uses a copious amount of oil and applies pressure in a circular clockwise motion on an unclothed recipient. The massage begins at the head and ends at the feet. Firm pressure is used on the limbs and light pressure is used on the neck, face, abdomen, and heart area. Pressure is used in the same direction as the body hair (along arterial flow). The recipient applies a powder and takes a warm bath 15 to 20 minutes after an Ayurvedic massage.

DEEP TISSUE

Deep tissue massage requires warming strokes and firm pressure to reach deeper layers of muscle and **fascia**. The therapist uses minimal lotion and incorporates arms and elbows to apply more pressure. It typically focuses on a specific area of muscle pain or tension to release adhesions, break down scar tissue, and realign muscle fibers.

MYOFASCIAL RELEASE

Myofascial release relaxes the fascia, which helps reduce tension and pain.

REFLEXOLOGY

Created 5,000 years ago by the Egyptians, **reflexology** associates specific points on the feet, hands, and ear with different body organs and systems. Pressure on these points is believed to influence the function of those organs and systems. Reflexology can be done clothed or unclothed, and no lotion is necessary.

SPORTS MASSAGE

Provided in sports clinics and on-site at sporting events (typically on covered tables with clothed athletes), pre-event **sports massage** uses energizing strokes, like rocking and shaking, and compressions to "wake up" an athlete's muscles and prepare them to compete. Post-event sports massage uses slower strokes to relax tired muscles and sedate the nervous system, allowing the athlete to "come down" from the stress of competition. Sports massage includes assisted stretching to heal sports injuries and improve range of motion.

SWEDISH MASSAGE

Developed in the early 1800s, Swedish massage is the premier Western form of touch therapy. It is typically done with the recipient unclothed under linens on a massage table. The therapist uses lotion to perform long, flowing strokes, like gliding (**effleurage**) and kneading (**petrissage**), and more targeted strokes, like friction, vibration, and tapping (**tapotement**). Pressure varies, usually starting light and ending firmer, with the goal of full-body relaxation.

THAI MASSAGE

Using the recipient's participation, **Thai massage** uses waves of gentle pressure and yoga-like stretching to gradually stretch the entire body and move energy along channels, or sen lines, that correspond to parts of the body like bones, muscles, blood, and nerves. Thai massage is energizing and relaxing, bringing a sense of physical and mental restoration. It is done on a floor mat with the recipient clothed to facilitate stretching.

TRIGGER POINT THERAPY

Trigger point therapy, developed by Dr. Janet Travell and Dr. David Simons in the 1970s, is used in medical massage clinics to address trigger points, which cause pain, complicate pain, and mimic pain. Trigger point therapy uses direct, focused pressure on these "hyperirritable spots in taut bands of muscle" to release them and restore blood flow, function, and strength to the muscle. The hallmark of trigger points is their classic **referral pattern**, which refers pain to other areas in the body when the trigger point is pressed. The pattern for each trigger point is the same for about 85 percent of people, making it easier to locate and relieve the source of the pain. These points are typically found at the junction where the nerve meets the muscle, so it is often called neuromuscular therapy.

THIS BOOK'S INTEGRATIVE APPROACH

Don't be overwhelmed by the many massage styles, strokes, and theories described here. The best practitioners integrate a wide variety of styles and strokes to customize the best massage for the recipient in every session; no two massages are ever the same.

As a medical massage therapist, I use a variety of techniques on a daily basis, depending on my patient's individual needs. I use the Eastern practice of rocking and shaking at the beginning and end of every massage and every body part, both to sedate the nervous system and to check how the body or limb is moving before and after my work. I use Swedish, Shiatsu, and sports massage strokes to warm up areas of the body before going in deeper with deep tissue, myofascial release, and trigger point therapy. During the massage, I incorporate Eastern acupressure points and hand, foot, and ear reflexology to enhance energy flow and address specific conditions I've noticed from listening to my patients' symptoms. And to finish, I do Thai and sports stretching to retrain the muscles on their appropriate length, and, as a yoga teacher and therapist, I recommend yoga poses to my patients to maintain the relief I accomplished.

The book in your hands right now will give you the best tools across all these disciplines and more for helping your partner with their specific ailments.

MASSAGE AT HOME

Doing massage at home has a lot of perks. In addition to saving money on massage therapy treatments, which currently range from $50 to $200 per hour, you will also be able to experience massage on a regular—maybe even daily—basis. And you'll save time traveling to and from a massage studio.

Instead of reaching for your pain pills, you will be able to use massage as pain relief whenever aches and pains trouble you. You can also use massage on demand to increase your circulation, relieve tension and sinus pressure, cut down cravings, and lessen symptoms of depression and anxiety.

If you are shy with strangers, giving yourself a massage or receiving one from a trusted family member or friend will allow you to enjoy the benefits of massage. You can feel more comfortable sharing what works and what doesn't, where you need pressure, and what feels good to you.

Most important, you can spend time with yourself. Quiet time is rare in our culture of chronic stress, and regular massage sessions for yourself or with a partner will become cherished time for mind-body connection and nonsexual intimacy and touch.

MANAGING EXPECTATIONS

As we've explored, massage affects the body in many ways. Your partner may have any number of physical sensations as you massage them. Most people enjoy the feeling of light and deep pressure and find themselves relaxing or even falling asleep—both are normal. They may also experience shivering, tremors, yawning, tears, goose bumps, or sweating, all signs that the body is switching out of fight-flight-or-freeze and into rest-and-digest (more about this on page 9), the relaxation response of the nervous system. As you release muscle tension, your partner may also feel quivering muscles, hot or cold sensations, and a sense of release in the specific area where you are working.

Your partner might also feel an emotional release: a sudden rush of powerful emotion, like grief, euphoria, anger, fear, or sadness, often brought on by pressure in an area of the body that was previously injured or tense during past trauma. Your partner may cry, laugh, yell, or go rigid. When you see them experiencing an emotional release, it is important to keep your hands **on** your partner and ask if they'd like to pause for a moment (grab a tissue, have some water, be alone, etc.), or if they'd like to continue. Reassure them that this is a normal reaction to massage; allow them to share if they feel open to it and to keep quiet if they need their privacy. Respect their vulnerability by staying present and by not offering advice, just support, as they work through their emotions.

After their massage, your partner may feel lightheaded or nauseous if they get up too quickly, so be sure to give them time to sit up slowly. Your partner may also need to use the bathroom after their session. Effective massage will result in their body feeling lighter, less restricted, and more freely movable. Hydrated tissue is healthy tissue, so encourage your partner to increase their water intake before and after their massage.

Massage will affect everyone (and every body) differently, so experiment with different styles and strokes to see what works best for your partner. Remember, massage is not a magic cure for disease and dysfunction, so don't be disappointed if your partner doesn't experience complete healing right away. Massage is a tool to manage symptoms and relieve pain, and it is more effective over time.

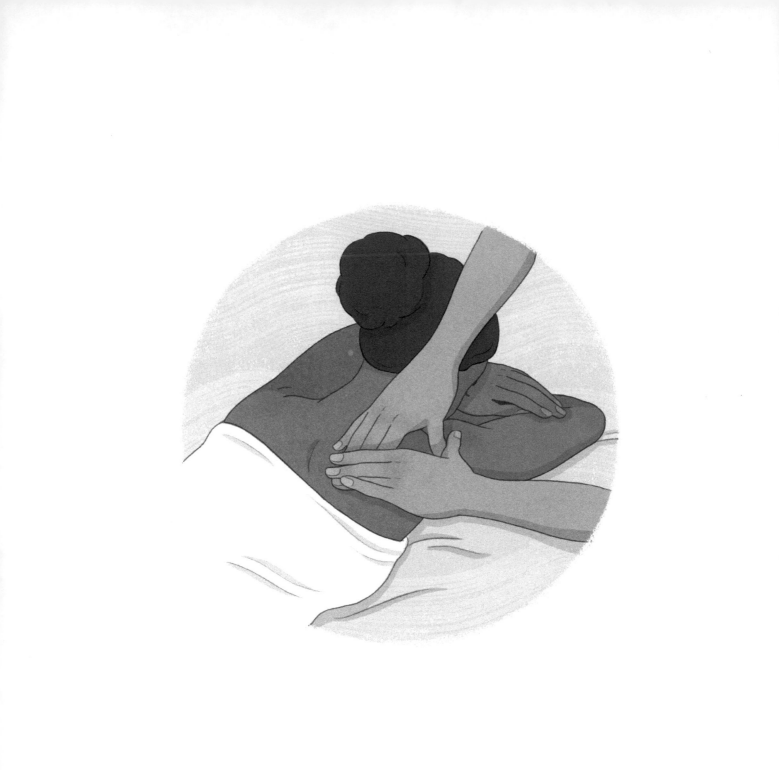

CHAPTER 2

The Basics of the Body

This chapter discusses the fundamental techniques you will be using in your massage, along with some basic anatomy and massage science to help you understand why massage is so beneficial for our bodies. You'll also learn things like how much pressure to apply and how to adjust your massage for recipients of all ages. You're probably anxious to get started, but the more you learn about how the body works, the better you'll be at giving an effective, healing massage.

MASSAGE ANATOMY

Let's go over some basic anatomy. Our movement and posture is made possible by three systems of the body: muscles, bones, and nerves. When these systems are working in proper alignment, we have ideal function, strength, and endurance. When they are out of alignment, we have dysfunction, weakness, and fatigue.

Muscles for movement are called **skeletal muscles**, as they attach to the bones in our skeleton. Skeletal muscles are arranged like bundles of sticks, with each "stick" being a muscle **fascicle**. Within each fascicle is another bundle of sticks, and each of those sticks is called a **muscle fiber**. These muscle fibers are made up of tiny protein filaments, which contract and relax when they receive signals from nerve endings attached to the muscles. A contraction will shorten the muscle, while a relaxation lengthens the muscle. When a muscle contracts, its attachment to a bone near a joint will cause that joint to flex or extend, resulting in movement. When the muscle relaxes, the bone should return to its original position.

Bones are the framework for our bodies. Bone is living, growing tissue made up of collagen (a protein that provides a soft framework) and calcium phosphate (a mineral that adds strength and density). Bones have a thick, dense outer layer and a light, spongy inner layer of **trabeculae**. These trabeculae are important for the strength of your bones, as they grow denser in response to the pull of the muscles on the bone. The more weight-bearing exercise you do, the stronger your bones become.

Joints are places in our bodies where two or more bones meet. Most of our joints allow for movement, which is called that joint's **range of motion**. In a joint, **ligaments** connect bone to bone and **tendons** connect muscle to bone. To lessen friction in a joint, **cartilage** covers the ends of the bones, and a sac called a **bursa** sits between the bones and other structures.

Nerves are the body's communication system, using bundles of long string-like nerve cells called **neurons** wrapped in fatty cells to rapidly conduct nerve impulses from the brain, spinal cord, skeletal muscles, and other body parts. Most of our skeletal muscles receive impulses from spinal nerves; they branch off from the spinal cord through spaces between the bones in the spine and carry messages along a specific area of the body known as a **dermatome**. When the nerve is affected anywhere along the

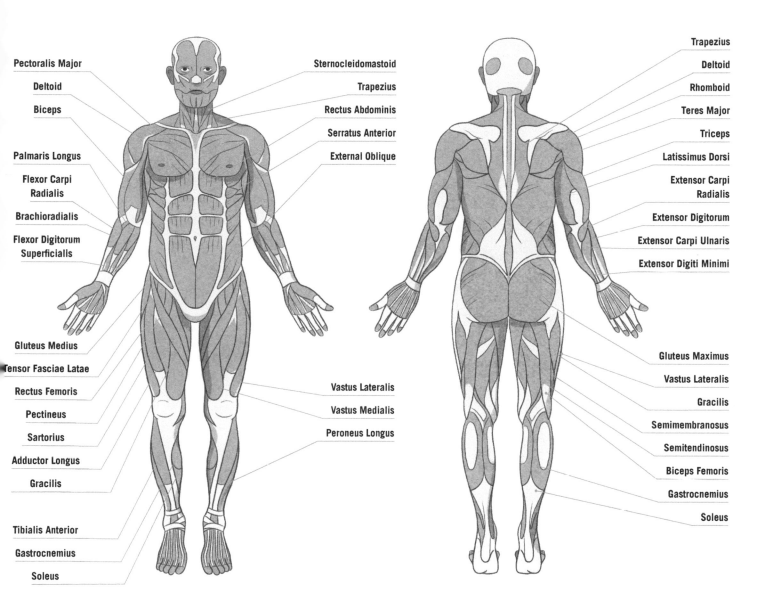

Pectoralis Major

Deltoid

Biceps

Palmaris Longus

Flexor Carpi
Radialis

Brachioradialis

Flexor Digitorum
Superficialis

Gluteus Medius

Tensor Fasciae Latae

Rectus Femoris

Pectineus

Sartorius

Adductor Longus

Gracilis

Tibialis Anterior

Gastrocnemius

Soleus

Sternocleidomastoid

Trapezius

Rectus Abdominis

Serratus Anterior

External Oblique

Vastus Lateralis

Vastus Medialis

Peroneus Longus

Trapezius

Deltoid

Rhomboid

Teres Major

Triceps

Latissimus Dorsi

Extensor Carpi
Radialis

Extensor Digitorum

Extensor Carpi Ulnaris

Extensor Digiti Minimi

Gluteus Maximus

Vastus Lateralis

Gracilis

Semimembranosus

Semitendinosus

Biceps Femoris

Gastrocnemius

Soleus

There are over 600 muscles in the body.
These are some of the main skeletal muscles
that are targeted during massage.

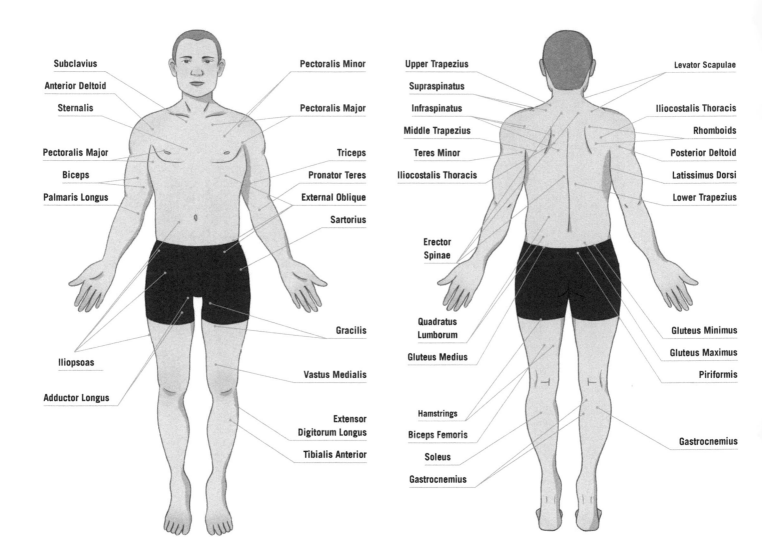

Subclavius
Anterior Deltoid
Sternalis
Pectoralis Major
Biceps
Palmaris Longus
Iliopsoas
Adductor Longus

Pectoralis Minor
Pectoralis Major
Triceps
Pronator Teres
External Oblique
Sartorius
Gracilis
Vastus Medialis
Extensor Digitorum Longus
Tibialis Anterior

Upper Trapezius
Supraspinatus
Infraspinatus
Middle Trapezius
Teres Minor
Iliocostalis Thoracis
Erector Spinae
Quadratus Lumborum
Gluteus Medius
Hamstrings
Biceps Femoris
Soleus
Gastrocnemius

Levator Scapulae
Iliocostalis Thoracis
Rhomboids
Posterior Deltoid
Latissimus Dorsi
Lower Trapezius
Gluteus Minimus
Gluteus Maximus
Piriformis
Gastrocnemius

Common Trigger Points

dermatome pathway, pain can also happen anywhere along the pathway. For example, an issue with the nerve in the upper back can cause forearm and hand pain, which makes it difficult to diagnose and treat.

Fascia is an interwoven system of connective tissue that holds together the entire body by coating your muscles, organs, and nerves and connecting muscles, bones, tendons, ligaments, and blood. Fascia is also made of collagen. When it is healthy, it allows muscle fibers and other tissues to slide, glide, and move freely. To understand the nature of fascia, picture an orange. When you peel the skin away, there is a thick layer of white, stringy flesh. This is like the thick layer of superficial fascia and fatty tissue just underneath your skin. The orange is also segmented, with each segment surrounded by a thin layer. This thin layer is like the deep fascia surrounding each muscle, fascicle, and muscle fiber. Finally, within each segment are tiny pieces of pulp, also surrounded by an ultra-thin layer. This layer is like the microscopic fascia surrounding your nerves, organs, and smaller structures.

Massage primarily works on muscles, but it also affects the function of bones, joints, nerves, and fascia.

Muscle tension is caused when a muscle contracts and does not release, which limits the flow of blood, oxygen, and nutrients to the area. Many factors contribute to lasting muscle tension, including stress, anxiety, dehydration, inadequate nutrition, traumatic injury, and overuse, repetitive use, or improper use of muscles during exercise and activities of daily life. Unhealthy fascia will dry out and become sticky in the area, limiting range of motion. Less movement may result in pain when the muscle is contracted again, which may in turn cause the muscle to spasm, leading to more pain. This is called the pain-spasm-pain cycle.

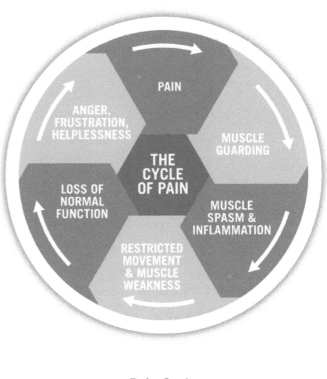

Pain Cycle

Massage increases circulation to an area of muscle tension, which returns the flow of oxygen and nutrients and allows contracted tissue to relax. Massage also warms and mobilizes the fascia, breaking the sticky connections that formed while the muscle was tense and creating a broader range of motion in the nearby joints. In injured and healed tissue, massage softens and realigns the scar tissue that formed in the area, which was hastily laid down like a pile of sticks to quickly close tissue gaps. When these issues are corrected, the muscle and fascia move freely, which reduces pain and improves joint function.

What Is a Knot?

Knots are areas in muscles that feel tight, dense, and sticky. The more dry and stuck it feels, the older the "knot" tends to be. There are generally three kinds of "knotted" tissue:

- **Adhesions:** This is where fascia has dried out, fuzzed up, and stuck together; these knots tend to feel sticky, long, and thin along the fiber of the muscle.

- **Scar tissue:** This describes previously injured areas where thick white fibers were quickly laid down in all directions to repair gaps in tissue. Think of a pile of sticks where once they had been an organized bundle; these knots tend to feel harder and less movable.

- **Trigger points:** These are areas where muscle contraction has cut off the flow of blood and nutrients to the area, resulting in microscopic contractions that don't let go; by the time you can feel these knots, there are thousands of them in one place.

No matter what kind of knotted tissue you find, massage science is simple—it breaks down scar tissue and increases circulation to the area, which releases trigger points, restores blood flow, and loosens fascia.

TYPES OF PRESSURE

Pressure is an important aspect of massage. Contrary to popular belief, you don't need a lot of pressure to do deep tissue massage. The body's layers of fascia and muscle are like the layers of an onion. A knife can slice through all the layers instantly, but it does long-term damage to the onion. In order to reach the center layers (the deepest layers) while keeping the onion whole, you need to melt and caramelize the outer layers. Massage, when done properly, warms and softens the layers one at a time, allowing access to each layer at its proper time. Given enough time and warming, all layers can be reached, no matter your pressure. So deep tissue massage is just massage that is done at the deeper layers.

> **TIP:**
> ▶ Deep tissue massage is different from firm pressure.

It is crucial that you apply enough pressure to affect the muscles, but not so much that you hurt your partner. In fact, too much pressure is the cause of bruising during a massage; when the pressure rises past your partner's pain threshold, it sends a message to the muscle to contract against the pressure, preventing it from releasing, which results in tissue damage and inflammation. Resist the urge to say, "No pain, no gain!" It's simply not true.

The most important component to your pressure is communication with your partner. If it feels painful to them, it is too much pressure. Plan to work on a pressure scale of 1 to 5, with 1 being feather-light, and 5 being so much pressure that they want to jump off the table. Aim for no higher than a 4, which is that "hurts so good" spot where your partner says, "Right there, but no more, please." Remember that the pressure scale changes depending on who you are massaging; something that feels like a 2 to one person may be a 5 to another. Always check in with your partner about the pressure any time you change the pressure, stroke, or location of your massage.

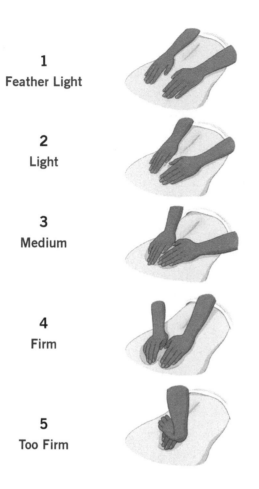

1
Feather Light

2
Light

3
Medium

4
Firm

5
Too Firm

- 1 to 2, light: feather-light to light, applying lotion, introducing touch, finishing the massage

- 3, medium: hands make a soft indent on the body, tissue is warming and moving underneath the hands

- 4, firm: hands make a deep indent on the body, tissue is pinned under pressure, your partner takes deep breaths, says, "Hurts so good;" "Right there, but no more, please"

- 5, too firm: "Stop," "Ouch," and nonverbal cues like flinching and sudden inhaling

10 FUNDAMENTAL TECHNIQUES

Here are the fundamental techniques you will use during massage. Part Two will refer to these movements, so flip back here any time you need a refresher. Remember these tips:

- Never massage across or on top of a bone. It hurts!
- Start with light pressure and gradually increase the pressure as the area warms.
- Always communicate with your partner about how the massage feels, asking for pressure on the scale from 1 to 5 each time you change the stroke, pressure, or location.

Acupressure

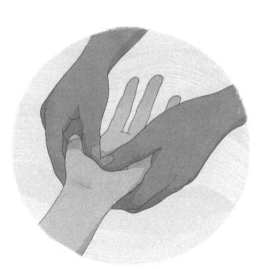

Acupressure changes the flow of energy at points on Traditional Chinese Medicine meridians, balances the overall flow in the body, and addresses specific conditions. I will recommend specific points for you to hold depending on the ailments.

1. Identify the point on your partner to hold according to their ailment.
2. Set your intention to move energy through that point.
3. Ask your partner to inhale, and match your breath to theirs.
4. With your thumb or pointer finger, lightly press straight down into the point as you and your partner exhale. Use a light pressure (1).
5. Release as your partner exhales or hold the point through a few breaths (at least 60 seconds).
6. Release when you feel it is time to move on.

Gliding (Effleurage)

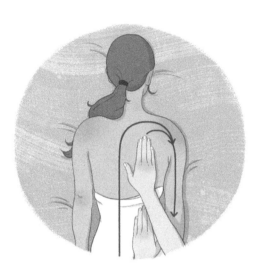

Gliding is a Swedish massage technique used to introduce your touch and warm the muscles. It stimulates the nervous system, increases lymph and blood flow, and stretches the tissues. Effleurage comes from the French word "effleurer," which means "to skim."

1. Apply lotion to one hand and rub your hands together to warm the lotion.
2. Place your hands palms down on the area to be massaged and allow your hands to follow the natural contours of the body.
3. Glide your hands along your partner's body with long, flowing strokes. Use a light to medium pressure (1 to 3).
4. Notice any areas of tension so you can return to them later.
5. Continue gliding as needed, increasing the pressure as the area warms up.

Kneading (Petrissage)

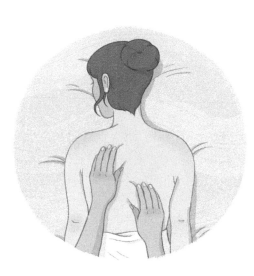

Kneading is a Swedish massage technique used to compress and release muscles. It improves the fascia's movement, increases lymph and blood flow, and relaxes muscles. Petrissage comes from the French word "pétrir," which means "to knead."

1. Once the area has been warmed by gliding (effleurage), move on to kneading.
2. Place the heels of your hands on the area and push away from you, one hand at a time. Use medium to firm pressure (3 to 4).
3. Reach across the body with your hands and pull back toward you, one hand at a time.
4. Form a C with your hands and pick up the area, wrapping the C around the muscle. Use both hands to shake the muscle, then slide the C along the muscle, one hand at a time, in opposite directions.

Friction

Friction strokes are small, firm movements applied across muscle fibers to separate adhesions, break down scar tissue, and stimulate healing and blood flow. Friction is typically used in myofascial release therapy in sports and medical clinics.

1. Warm the area with gliding and kneading before using friction strokes. Use medium to firm pressure (3 to 4).
2. Find a taut band of muscle tension that resists your pressure.
3. Using stacked fingers or supported thumbs, press the pads of the fingers into that band of muscle tension perpendicularly (so your pressure is directed into and across the band).
4. Firmly and quickly press the fingers across the band one hand at a time, alternating strokes along the muscle in one direction.
5. Using stacked hands, make circles with the pads of the fingers as you press into the band and move along the muscle in one direction.
6. Once you feel the muscle release (the band softening), use gliding strokes to "warm out" and relax the muscle before moving on.

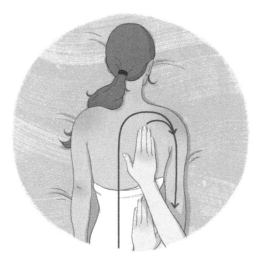 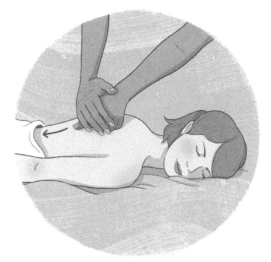

Trigger Point Therapy

Trigger point therapy is used in medical massage to address trigger points, which cause pain, complicate pain, and mimic pain. It uses direct, focused pressure on these hyperirritable spots to release them and restore blood flow, function, and strength to the muscle.

1. Find spots that cause and/or refer pain when pressed. This sensation indicates a trigger point is present in the muscle.
2. Warm the area until it is pink and warm to the touch using gliding, kneading, or friction strokes. Use a light to firm pressure (1 to 4).
3. With your stacked fingers, stacked hands, or supported thumb, press into the spot that causes or refers pain. Ask your partner to give you a number from 1 to 5 on the pressure scale based on what they are feeling from your pressure.
4. Hold the pressure until the number decreases to 1 or 2, and then release.
5. Once you feel the trigger point release (the spot quivers or softens, and the referral pain decreases), use gliding strokes to "warm out" and relax the muscle before moving on.

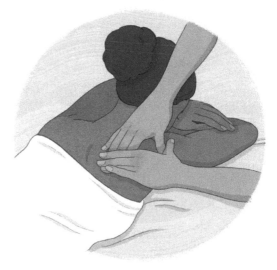

Percussion (Tapotement)

Percussion is a Swedish massage technique used to stimulate the nervous system and lymph and blood flow. Tapotement comes from the French word "tapoter," which means "to tap or drum." Do not use percussion over bones, and don't use it on muscles after athletic activity, either, as it may cause cramping and spasms.

1. With your hands facing each other, either open or in soft fists, lightly and quickly strike the area with the sides of your hands. Use a light pressure (1 to 2).

2. With your hands cupped and facing downward, lightly and quickly strike the area with hands.
3. With your hands facing downward, lightly tap your fingertips on the area.

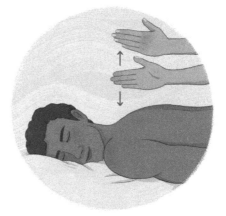

Vibration

Vibration is a massage technique that lightly shakes an area of your partner's body using vibration you produce in your hands and arms. It can soothe irritated nerves, increase blood and lymph flow, and relax the muscles. Use it sparingly, since it uses muscle tension in your body to create the vibrations.

1. Stack your hands with one palm on top of the other and straighten your arms, pressing your hands firmly into your partner's body. Use a light-medium pressure (1 to 3).

2. Tense your arm muscles to create a fine, trembling movement that transfers into your partner's body.

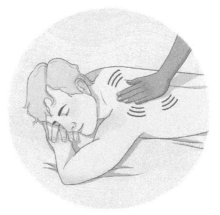

Feathering

Feathering is a massage technique that softly stimulates and relaxes the nervous system, much like stroking a cat.

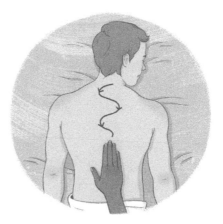

1. Start with one hand, your palm down and fingers together. Lightly and smoothly stroke down the area with your fingertips, closely followed by your other hand.
2. Alternate your hands repeatedly for 1 to 3 minutes.

Stretching

Stretching is an Eastern and Western technique used in Thai, Shiatsu, sports, and medical massage. Stretching is typically used at the end of a Western massage session to integrate the bodywork into the muscles' memory. By stretching the newly lengthened muscle, you remind the muscle how long it can be and help retain that length.

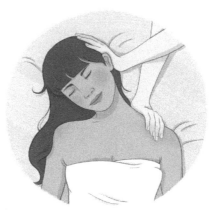

1. Ensure that the tissue is warm before stretching.
2. To stretch a muscle, move the two ends of the muscle away from each other by applying firm pressure to one end in the opposite direction from the other end.

3. To increase the stretch, pin down one end of the muscle as you move the other end away.

Rocking and Shaking

Rocking and shaking is an Eastern massage technique used to sedate the nervous system, much like rocking a crying baby or sitting in a rocking chair. It is also used in Western massage sessions as a warming tool to evaluate an area's movement and tension, and as a sports massage technique to release the muscles before and after an athletic event. Dr. Janet Travell, personal physician to President Kennedy, actually prescribed him a rocking chair to alleviate his chronic lower-back pain!

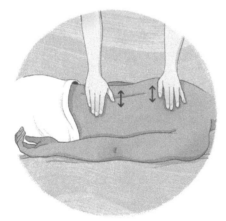

Rocking and shaking is done along the spine and the limbs. The pace may be fast or slow, depending on your partner's rhythm.

1. To rock and shake the spine, face your partner and place one hand palm down at the base of the neck, and the other palm down at the base of the spine.
2. To rock and shake the leg, face your partner and place one hand in a soft fist at the side of the hip, and the other hand palm down at the calf.
3. To rock and shake the arm, face your partner and place one hand in a soft fist at the side of the shoulder, and the other hand palm down at the forearm.
4. Lightly press down and move your hands away and then toward you at a pace that moves the whole spine, arm, or leg.
5. Once a rhythm has been established, continue to roll back and forth as you move your hands along your partner's entire body, looking for tension and sticky spots in the rhythm.

BODY MECHANICS OF THE MASSAGE THERAPIST

It is important to protect your body when you are giving a massage to keep you from ending up with aches and pains of your own. Rather than wearing out your fingers and thumbs, massage like a pro by using stacked joints, to transfer your body weight into your hands.

To provide the best pressure, stand or kneel in a lunge facing your partner on a table, bed, or chair. The back foot or knee in your lunge provides the push-off point to transfer your weight. Your spine stays straight (no bending at the waist). Extend your arms in front of you so your shoulders, elbows, and wrists are in a straight line (without locking out the joints). We call these stacked joints. With your hands connected to your partner's body, push off your back foot or knee, keeping your hip and spine stacked in line with your back foot, and the arm joints stacked in front of you. Your pressure should travel into your partner. Bring your back foot or knee toward your partner to decrease your pressure, and move it away to increase the pressure.

TIP:

▶ The deeper your lunge, the firmer the pressure.

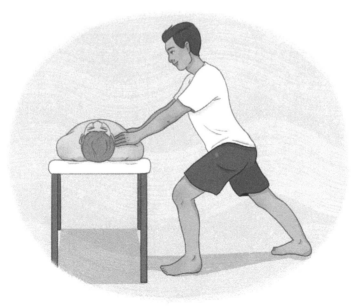

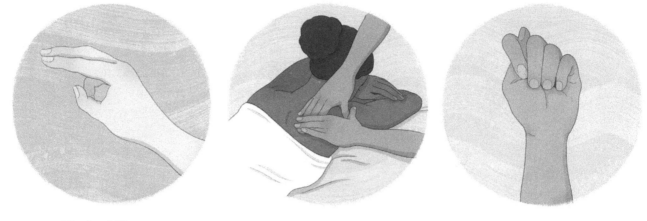

Stacked Fingers   **Stacked Hands**   **Supported Thumb**

Use healthy hand positions to keep from hurting your finger, thumb, and wrist joints. For stacked fingers, stack your middle finger on top of your pointer finger. For stacked hands, place one hand over the other with the pointer, middle, and ring fingers overlapping. When stacking, the bottom hand or finger is the tool, and the top hand or finger applies the pressure (which in turn comes from the back foot or knee). For supported thumbs, keep your thumbs outside a closed fist and use the fist to reinforce your thumb pressure. You can also support your thumb between the pointer and middle finger of a closed fist (like the "got your nose" joke).

Energy and Grounding

Massage also works on an energetic level. As we mentioned earlier, Eastern practices like Traditional Chinese Medicine place enormous importance on the flow of energy within the body. Massage therapists in the East and West agree that an energy exchange takes place when we touch another person with intent to heal.

An important aspect of massage is staying grounded and intentional with your touch. Grounding is a technique of preparing to give or receive a massage by letting go of your own stress and being present in the moment with your partner. Grounding allows you to set your intention for your massage, increase your focus, and improve the benefits of the massage for your partner.

Since your partner will release energy as their muscles release, you want to provide a channel for that release, but you do not want to keep any of their energy. You also want to make sure that anything you are dealing with emotionally or physically doesn't become a part of your partner's experience. Energetically, it is important to take nothing with you once your session is done, and to leave nothing with your partner.

Here are a few examples of ways for you to stay grounded during your session:

- Before you start, take a few deep breaths with your eyes closed.
- Tell yourself that you are here for your partner, and you are leaving your own issues at the door.
- Stay present with your partner, noticing their breath, movement, and words.
- Focus on the feel of their muscles beneath your hands.
- Visualize your connection with the earth. For example, picture yourself growing roots like a tree and drawing energy from the earth.
- Visualize your energy joining with your partner's energy. Picture your partner's energy as a pool of water, and as you begin the massage, you step into that pool.
- As you end your massage, take a few deep breaths with your eyes closed. Picture the end of your visualization (drawing up roots, stepping out of the pool, etc.). Take a moment to remove your hands from your partner and thank them for allowing you to give them a massage.

SPECIAL CONSIDERATIONS FOR ALL

Depending on your partner, there may be special considerations to take into account (in addition to the Contraindications on page 6). Read through the list to see if your partner falls into any of these categories and adjust your massage to include these special techniques.

Self-Massage

The biggest challenge when massaging yourself is body mechanics, since it is difficult to protect your joints when you can't use the weight transfer from your lunge to get good pressure (see Chapter 3). Luckily for you, there are some tricks for hitting a spot you really need to get to.

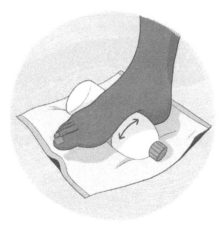

FROZEN WATER BOTTLE
This tool is great for areas with intense pain and inflammation, like the sole of the foot or the **perineum** (between the genitals and the anus).

1. Place the water bottle under the area with a towel or clothing between the bottle and the skin. Use the easiest position to apply pressure to the spot, like sitting down for the perineum or standing up for the sole of the foot.
2. Use gentle pressure or a rocking motion to apply cold until the area is cold to the touch and pain decreases, which is usually after a few minutes.

TENNIS AND LACROSSE BALLS

Use tennis balls for softer pressure and lacrosse balls for firmer pressure. A ball inside a sock will make it easier to move the ball once it's in place. These balls can be used anywhere on the body to produce focused pressure, similar to trigger point therapy, or moving pressure, like friction.

1. Lean against the ball on a wall or lie on the floor with the ball underneath you, placing the ball under your trigger point or muscle tension.

2. With your knee(s) bent, use your feet against the wall or floor to move around, or allow your body weight to soften over the ball.

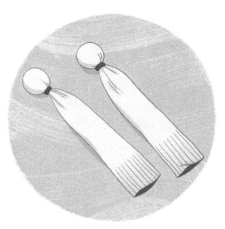

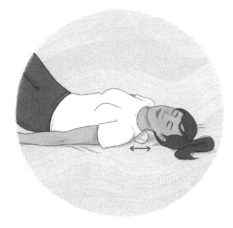

Modern Tools for Self-Massage

FOAM ROLLER, $10–$20

Many foam rollers exist, from simple pool noodles to fancy "trigger point" foam rollers with ridges and nubs. Whichever you choose, use it for light rolling to warm and loosen superficial fascia. Foam rollers are not appropriate for deep work, as their broad surface will cause bruising before deep tissue release occurs. Foam rolling is beneficial for tension in large areas of the body, like the legs, hips, and back muscles.

1. Lie on the floor face up and place the foam roller under your back or glutes.
2. Bend your knees and use your feet flat on the floor to roll over the roller.
3. On your side, place the roller under your hips or IT band and use a side plank or push-up position with your hands to roll over the roller.
4. On your stomach, place the roller under your quads and use your hands in push-up or plank position to roll forward and back.

MASSAGE HOOK, $20–$40

This tool comes in many shapes and sizes and is designed to give you leverage, allowing you to increase the pressure without hurting yourself. Be careful with pressure, since most of these hooks are made of plastic. This hook is best for acupressure points or trigger points that you need to hold but can't reach.

1. After warming an area, hook into a trigger point or tense area, starting with light pressure.
2. Use trigger point therapy to release the area, holding pressure on the spot and moving the long arm of the hook up, down, or to the side to change the pressure.
3. Hold acupressure spots in the area with light pressure.

TENS UNIT, $15 TO $200

A transcutaneous electrical nerve stimulation (TENS) unit sends low-voltage electrical currents through adhesive electrode pads on the skin, blocking nerve signals and thus relieving pain. TENS units have been shown to provide both temporary and permanent pain relief, depending on the condition. They can be used to address specific muscle tension, muscle cramping, and trigger points.

1. Use your TENS unit as often as you need it, for up to 15 minutes. Follow your unit's instructions to place the electrode pads where they will provide the best relief for your pain.

Seniors

Older people deal with stiff muscles, limited movement, and chronic pain. They are more likely to have conditions that are contraindicated for massage, so read the list in chapter 1 (page 6) with your partner carefully. Here are some other things to consider when massaging this population:

- Your massage should be shorter than the average session, usually no longer than 30 minutes.
- Their skin has less moisture and is more likely to bruise and tear, so use lighter pressure, gentler strokes, and milder stretching.
- You may need to help your partner get undressed and dressed, adjust your surface so they can get on and off more easily, or adapt your massage to work on your partner in a wheelchair or with whatever assistive device they may use.

- Use feathering strokes along the spine, arm, hand, or foot to sedate your partner's nervous system and alleviate symptoms of depression and anxiety.
- Give a full-body Swedish massage at light to medium pressure, using gliding strokes on the back, arms, legs, hands, and feet. Finish with gentle thumb strokes on the face and ears.
- Use a reflexology chart to press points on the hands, feet, and ears to relieve symptoms in a corresponding area.

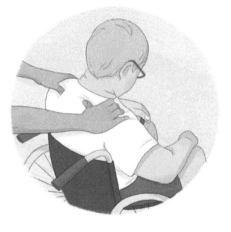

Babies and Children

Touch is an essential part of a child's development. Nurturing touch encourages growth in all aspects of a child's life. Just as in adults, massage can improve quality of sleep, reduce aggressive behavior, relieve constipation, and even enhance self-esteem and body image. For children dealing with extraordinary stressors, research has shown that massage can help with autism, cancer, cerebral palsy, and mental health conditions, like depression and anxiety caused by death, divorce, illness, homelessness, and more.

- Most massage on babies and children is done fully clothed.
- If the child has parents who are not you, be sure you have their consent to give their child a massage.
- Babies and children are especially vulnerable during a massage, so ensure that you have their permission to give them one. If the child cannot speak, watch for nonverbal cues like pulling away, shallow breathing, or muscle tightness, all of which show that the child is afraid or unwilling to participate.
- Babies and younger children are likely to need very short sessions—less than 15 to 20 minutes—due to their short attention spans.
- Allow the child to control the pressure. Babies and children are more likely than adults to test different levels of pressure, mostly to see if you will actually respond to their requests. Children are also likely to be more demanding than adults. They will remember exactly what they liked before and randomly request those strokes, interrupting your flow. To build trust, respond each and every time they ask you to change something.

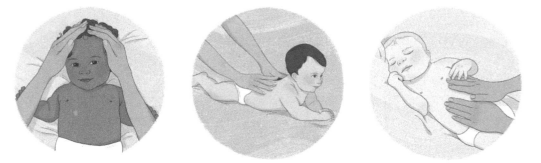

Prenatal

In addition to the typical benefits, prenatal massage has been shown to improve labor outcomes and newborn health, regulate hormone levels for more relaxation and less stress, reduce swelling and nerve pain, and improve sleep. Gentle massage is safe during all three trimesters of pregnancy, except if contraindicated.

- Massage is contraindicated during pregnancy if it is a high-risk pregnancy, or if there is pregnancy-induced high blood pressure, preeclampsia, severe swelling, or preterm labor.

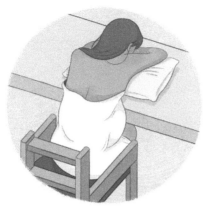

- Deep tissue massage and firm pressure is contraindicated during pregnancy. Since a pregnant person is already carrying up to 50 percent more blood than before the pregnancy, increasing the circulation with deep tissue work and firm pressure is likely to cause lightheadedness, dizziness, nausea, and vomiting.
- Avoid massaging the belly. Also, avoid the pressure points behind the ankle on both sides, which are believed to induce uterine contractions, and the pressure point where the neck meets the shoulder, which is believed to raise blood pressure.
- Avoid essential oils like oregano, nutmeg, peppermint, thyme, basil, clary sage, and rosemary, as they are believed to induce uterine contractions.

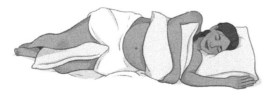

- Safe positions include on the back until 22 weeks (use a small wedge under the right hip), side-lying at any time (though the left side is safest for longer periods of time), and seated in a chair at any time during the pregnancy (have your partner lean forward on a table with a pillow under their head and arms). It is not safe to lay face down, even on a table with a hole for the pregnant belly, since it puts pressure on the abdomen or allows it to dangle, stretching the uterine ligaments.
- When side-lying, make sure your partner is on their right side for no more than 20 to 30 minutes at a time. However, lying on the left side is okay for up to 60 minutes.
- Have a lot of extra pillows and towels to use as bolsters to get them comfortable on the massage table.
- Your partner is likely to fall asleep during massage. Not only is that normal, but it should be encouraged!
- Use feathering strokes along the spine for up to 3 minutes to sedate the nervous system and allow rest.
- Give a full-body Swedish massage at light to medium pressure, using gliding strokes on the back, arms, legs, hands, and feet. Finish with gentle thumb strokes on the face and ears.
- Pay special attention to the neck, lower back, legs, and feet, and anywhere your partner requests (except the belly).

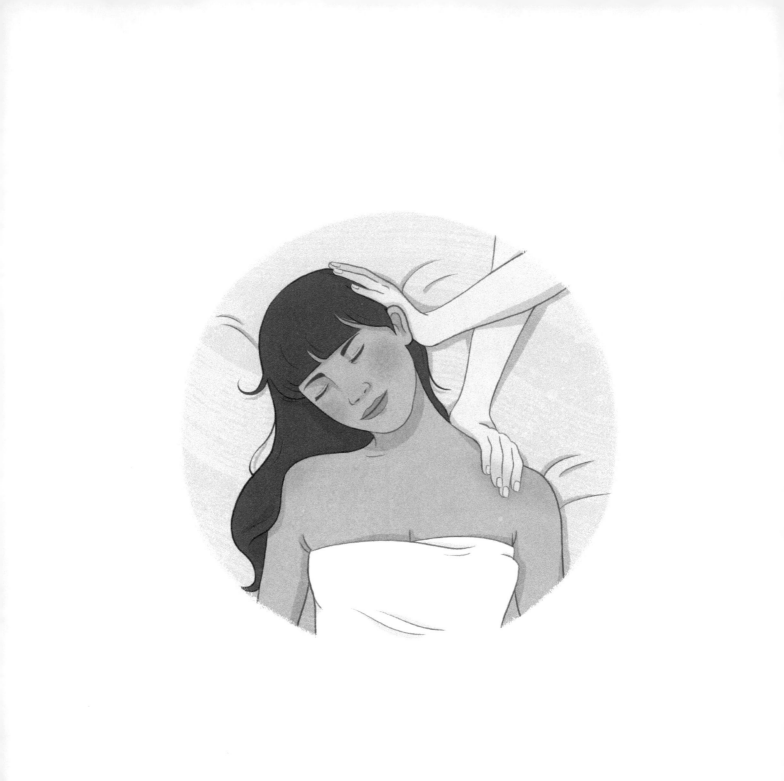

CHAPTER 3

Preparing for Massage

Getting started with massage is easy—all you need are your hands! That said, it is important to set up a safe and comfortable massage space for you and your partner. It's important to consider your communication, clothing, environment, and accessories before starting your massage. These aspects of your massage will set the stage for a truly relaxing experience for both of you.

BEST PRACTICES

Massage is an intense experience, for both the giver and receiver. For a safe and enjoyable experience, avoiding injury for you and your partner, there are some safety guidelines to follow. Many of these topics are covered in detail in chapters 1 and 2, but this list is a handy reference as you prepare to move on to the techniques in part 2.

1. Before anything else, read the contra-indications for massage (page 6) to ensure that massage is a safe option for your partner. If modifications are needed, do research and have your partner check with their doctor before proceeding.

2. Have open, honest communication with your partner about boundaries (physical or otherwise), pressure, clothing, and the massage environment.

3. Agree to a drug-free and alcohol-free space before and during the massage, for both you and your partner.

4. Ensure that your hands and arms are clean and sanitized before you begin, as well as the massage surface, linens, and massage accessories.

5. Stay grounded during the massage to protect your energy and your partner's experience.

6. Use proper body mechanics to protect your own joints and muscles.

7. Respect your partner's requests during the massage: "Stop," "Less pressure," "No more in that spot"—they are in charge of their massage. They are vulnerable on the table, so give them the power and create a safe space for their massage.

8. After deep tissue massage, wait at least three days before massaging the same area again, giving the body time to integrate the work accomplished in the massage and preventing injury and inflammation in the area.

9. Don't do anything that makes you or your partner uncomfortable.

YOU AND YOUR PARTNER

In order to give an effective massage, there are a few important things that must exist between you and your partner: consent, trust, and communication.

Consent
Consent is important in massage because it clarifies expectations before anyone is unclothed on the table. It allows you to set healthy boundaries with your partner, and it gives your partner the power to control

what goes on during the massage, including when to stop.

What your consent means: You are offering your partner the gift of your massage. You should not give a massage when you are uncomfortable or not feeling well.

What your partner's consent means: Your partner needs to be in the right frame of mind to receive a massage. They should not receive a massage unless they feel comfortable, safe, and prepared to experience massage.

If you and your partner want to be sure you understand each other, you can agree to follow the best practices on page 42 or develop your own personal guidelines to ensure that both of you have consented to the massage.

Trust

In order for your partner to allow their muscles and emotions to release, they must know they can be vulnerable with you and trust your touch and your emotional support during your massage. Create a safe space for your partner by respecting their boundaries, maintaining a clean environment, and offering support (but not advice) during your massage.

Here are some tips to build trust between you and your partner in this setting. It's important to practice these skills even when your partner isn't with you, so it becomes part of your character:

- Prioritize your connection with your partner above being right or winning an argument. In every interaction, ask yourself, "How would I behave if my connection with my partner were the most important thing to me right now?"
- Practice honesty and vulnerability in all aspects of your relationship with your partner.
- Be genuine and authentic at all times.
- Celebrate your partner's differences from you.
- Respect your partner's privacy.
- Show empathy for your partner's struggles.
- Don't say negative things about your partner, to their face or behind their back.
- Support your partner's life choices— be their greatest cheerleader.

Communication

Communication is a two-way street in every relationship, and it's no different during massage. In fact, it's essential for your partner's safety, comfort, and healing process. You must be willing to listen to your partner, respect their requests, and receive their feedback about your touch. Your partner must also be willing to ask for what they need, speak up when they are uncomfortable, and give honest feedback about what feels good and what doesn't work for them.

To protect your partner, check in with them every time you change your pressure, stroke, or location during the massage (particularly in the first few sessions). Try asking questions like:

- "How does that feel?"
- "Do you like that stroke?"
- "I saw you flinch—does that feel okay?"
- And, of course, "On the pressure scale from 1 to 5, what number would you give my pressure here?"

If healthy feedback is a new concept for your partner, have them try a praise sandwich, giving you two compliments around each suggestion they have for you after the massage. Here's what this will look like:

- "I liked . . ."
- "I would have liked it better if . . ."
- "I liked . . ."

If your partner struggles to identify their needs in real life (and you have a healthy foundation for communication), encourage them to focus on their thoughts and feelings during the massage and practice voicing their thoughts about pressure, speed, and location: "That feels good," "More pressure there," "I don't like that," etc. As they practice this during a massage, it will come easier in real life.

Unclothed or Not?

It's up to your partner to decide whether to receive massage unclothed or clothed. They should decide based on their comfort level with you and their personal preference during a massage. If they are unable to relax while unclothed, have them wear light sportswear on top of a sheet, or a layer of underclothing while draped under a sheet. You can keep everything covered with the sheet except the part you're currently working on.

If your partner decides to stay clothed, some techniques requiring lotion to glide will not be possible during the massage, including gliding (effleurage) and kneading (petrissage). However, some techniques are only done clothed, including acupressure, Shiatsu, Thai, and stretching in sports massage, so your partner can still receive a wonderful massage.

The remaining techniques can be done clothed or unclothed: trigger point therapy, friction, percussion (tapotement), vibration, feathering, compression, and rocking and shaking.

No matter what your partner decides, honor their decision and do not ask them to change their mind unless you feel uncomfortable with their choice. Keep the line of communication open so you both feel comfortable and safe.

CREATING A RELAXED ENVIRONMENT

A safe and comfortable environment for massage sets the stage for a relaxing massage experience for you and your partner. There are many factors to consider, including location, atmosphere, equipment, accessories, and your own preparation. This section will help you choose the right elements to create the perfect massage environment for your and your partner.

Location

Choose the right location for your massage so that your partner can relax and you have enough room to protect your joints. Ensure that the space you choose has enough room for you to do a deep lunge (standing or kneeling) so that you can transfer your weight into your hands (as discussed in chapter 2).

Flat surfaces. If your partner will be lying down, choose a flat surface with full access on one side. If you give massages regularly, it is worthwhile to invest in a massage table. If you use a couch or a bed, have your partner lie close to the edge—you'll get better pressure that way. Work one full side, then have your partner switch to give you access to the other side. If your partner is lying on the floor, have them use a soft mat for padding. Use a kneeling lunge for giving massage on the floor. For light strokes, you can kneel on both knees and rise up to deliver your strokes.

Chairs. Choose a sturdy chair with a back and no arms. Have your partner sit backward and rest their head and arms on the back of the chair (preferably with a pillow for comfort). Use a standing lunge to massage the head, neck, and shoulders, and a kneeling lunge to massage the lower back, hips, and legs.

Atmosphere

The atmosphere makes a difference in your partner's ability to relax and your ability to stay grounded and focus on your partner. Take a few moments to set the right mood for your massage with the following elements:

Lighting. Choose dim lighting. You'll want to be able to see what you're doing, but a darker room allows their nervous system to relax.

Music. Music provides an escape on the table, giving you and your partner something to focus on to drift into a meditative state. For a relaxing massage, choose soft instrumental music with a slow beat.

Aromatherapy. Smell is a powerful memory trigger; take advantage with a scented candle or oil diffuser. Essential oils may also have healing properties, so you can diffuse certain oils to have a desired effect.

Cleanliness. It's important to massage in a tidy environment. Physical clutter overloads your senses, making you feel stressed and impairing your ability to think creatively. Spend a few minutes clearing the clutter away—you don't want to trip over anything as you massage.

Temperature. Set the temperature in the room at mid 70s—warm enough for your partner, who might cool down on the table, and cool enough for you, since you will be moving and sweating as you massage your partner.

EQUIPMENT AND ACCESSORIES

You don't need to spend a lot of money to get started—all you need is your hands—but investing in some of the following products can upgrade the quality of your massage.

Lubricants

Normal body lotion is intended to sink into the skin, while massage products are designed to stay on the skin's surface longer to allow to you glide as you massage. These are all available online for $10 to $20 for a pump bottle:

Massage oil. Oil has maximum glide with a small amount. Oil is the least absorbent and the most likely to stain your linens.

Massage lotion. Lotion typically has enough glide for Swedish strokes, with some friction for deeper work. Lotion absorbs into the skin more easily than oil.

Massage gel. Gel glides like oil and absorbs into the skin like lotion.

Massage creme. The thickest (and most expensive) of the lubricants, creme has a lot of friction for deep tissue work in a particular area. It absorbs into the skin like lotion.

Warming oil. This warms between your hands, making it easier to warm your partner's body. It acts like an oil and is good for both gliding strokes and deep tissue work.

Cooling sprays and gels. Used on a sore area after massage to provide extra pain relief (like using ice).

Linens and Bolsters

Depending on your massage surface, you may need to use linens and bolsters.

Table, bed, couch, or floor. Use a bottom sheet, a top sheet, and a blanket. Have your partner lie down under the top sheet and blanket, and tuck a bolster under their knees or ankles. During the massage, uncover only the part you are massaging, tucking the sheet and blanket around it for safety and comfort. To keep your partner comfortable while lying down, tuck something under their knees (when they are face up) or ankles (when they are face down). This prop takes the pressure off their lower back and allows for greater comfort during the massage. You can use a massage bolster, pillow, or rolled-up towel. If they have chronic lower-back pain, they may need an extra bolster layer (or some prefer no bolster at all).

Chair. No linens are needed since your partner will be clothed; just make sure you have a pillow or towel for their head and arms to rest on.

AROMATHERAPY AND MASSAGE

Essential oils and aromatherapy are a great way to add benefits to your massage. You can use a scented candle, diffuse oils in the room, or add oils to your lotion and apply them directly to the body.

There is little scientific evidence to support the health benefits of essential oils, but as with massage, that is no reason to ignore them. The following benefits are asserted by top essential oil companies and reported by millions of satisfied users; however, they are not intended to diagnose or treat any medical condition. Try them out for yourself and see how they affect you and your partner.

> **APPLICATION TIP:**
>
> ▶ When you use lotion with essential oils added, rub your hands together and wave them near your partner's nose to let them enjoy the scent.

Using Essential Oils

Always dilute essential oils in a carrier oil or lotion before applying them to the body. You can premake bottles with diluted oils for easy access during your massage, including droppers and rollers. Carrier oils for massage include almond oil, fractionated coconut oil, jojoba oil, sunflower oil, or apricot kernel oil. Be sure to check with your partner for allergies before using essential oils.

With children, it's important to avoid using stronger essential oils, even if they are diluted. Avoid birch, rosemary, wintergreen, and eucalyptus with children under the age of 12. For children under six, also stay away from oils derived from herbs and spices (like sage, marjoram, peppermint, cinnamon, nutmeg, etc.). The caution list is much longer for children under two, so do your research before using essential oils with younger children and babies. There are many oils that are safe with children over 12, including lavender, orange, geranium, chamomile, and more.

Here are six must-have essential oils for your massage collection:

Cypress: Cypress has a grounding and stimulating effect on the emotions, so it is often used during times of transition or loss. It creates an uplifting and energizing atmosphere. When applied to the body, it helps improve the appearance of oily skin and energizes the body and mind.

Eucalyptus: Eucalyptus refreshes the environment and stimulates the mind, creating a perfect atmosphere for study, meditation, or exercise. On the body, it cleanses and refreshes the skin with a tingling sensation and promotes feelings of clear breathing and open airways.

Geranium: Geranium creates a peaceful, spiritual atmosphere and helps calm nerves and lessen feelings of stress. When applied to the body, it promotes beautiful, radiant skin. It is also a natural bug repellent.

Lavender: Lavender promotes feelings of calm and fights nervous tension. It has balancing properties that calm the mind and body and promote peaceful sleep. It cleanses and soothes the skin, including blemishes, sunburn, and the effects of aging.

Peppermint: Peppermint creates a stimulating, focused atmosphere for daily tasks. When applied to the body, it creates a cool, tingling sensation, soothing sore and tired muscles.

Wintergreen and birch: Wintergreen and birch have the same main component, salicylate, which has a soothing and stimulating effect. It warms the tissues and relieves tired and sore muscles. **Safety note!** Wintergreen is highly toxic in concentrated essential oil form. Any massage blend should only use less than 2 percent wintergreen, and never, ever ingest it orally.

APPLYING HEAT AND ICE

As you massage your partner, you may find that using heat or ice is recommended. This section describes how to use hot and cold therapy to help your partner recover and heal from injuries, muscle cramps, and chronic pain. If both methods are recommended, alternate heat and ice on the affected area, always starting with heat and ending with ice.

Applying Heat
Heat naturally relaxes the muscles. It has a sedative effect on tense or sore muscles, which makes it perfect for preparing your partner for massage. You can use hot towels, hot stones, or even lotions and oils that heat up between your hands. You can also have your partner take a hot shower or hot bath (with Epsom salts for added relief) to warm up their body before you give them a massage. When using heat, be sure to do the following:

- Apply heat to any part of your partner's body that feels tense or sore.
- Make sure that whatever you put on your partner is tolerable to your own hands.
- Always check in with your partner while applying heat—when you first put it on and also 2 to 3 minutes later, as it can get too warm while it sits on the skin.

HOT TOWELS

1. Soak a towel under the faucet, wring it out, fold it into quarters, and microwave it until warm, usually 1 to 30 seconds right before using it on your partner.
2. Lay the towel on your partner's body (folded at least in half, if not more, to fit in the area).
3. Leave the towel on your partner and work another area as the towel warms up that spot. Remove the towel once it reaches body temperature.

HOT STONES

1. Don't use just any stone! Hot stones for massage are typically dark in color and made of basalt (lava rock), which holds heat really well. You can buy an affordable set online.
2. Place the stones in a pot and fill the pot with water so it covers the stones.

3. Heat the water over low temperature on the stove; if you have a temperature gauge, it's safe to heat stones up to 450 degrees Fahrenheit. It is important to heat hot stones slowly so they do not crack—do not use the microwave for this. Do this step at least an hour before the massage.
4. Right before you use the stones during your massage, use tongs or a skimmer to pull them out of the pot and onto a towel on the counter. If they are too hot for you to touch, you can also put them in a bowl of water to cool for a few seconds.
5. Place a towel or blanket on your partner's body where you want to put the stones. This layer will protect their body from being burned as the stones sit on their skin.
6. Choose the stone you will use for the area. You can use any size stone that fits. Big stones are great for large muscles, and small stones work well in tiny places (like between the toes or behind the neck).
7. Place the stones on your partner's body and cover the stones with another towel or blanket. The stones will keep their heat longer if they are covered.
8. Leave the stones in place to heat up the muscles, and massage a different part of your partner's body.

9. Take the stones off when they reach body temperature; your partner's body will stay warm even after the stones have been removed.
10. Wash your stones well with soapy water after using them.

LOTIONS AND OILS THAT HEAT UP

1. Put a small amount in your hands and rub them together briskly. The friction creates heat, which the lotion or oil enhances with menthol or other ingredients.
2. Use your heated hands to massage your partner's body, which will warm their muscles and skin faster.
3. Don't touch your eyes afterward!

Applying Ice

Inflammation occurs when an area is injured and white blood cells rush to the area to begin the healing process. Inflamed areas are typically swollen, soft, and squishy, and possibly painful, red, or warm to the touch. Cold naturally slows circulation and prevents additional swelling in an inflamed area, protecting your partner from secondary injury due to excessive swelling (which cuts off blood flow and prevents healing and waste removal from an injury site). Cold also numbs the area temporarily, relieving nerve pain. You can use cold or frozen towels, ice cubes, or even cooling lotions and oils. When using cold, be sure to do the following:

- Always use cold or ice after all other massage techniques in a sore or painful area, including stretching.
- Check in with your partner while applying cold or ice, both when you first put it on and also 2 to 3 minutes later, as it can get too cold as you apply it to the skin.
- Your partner may feel a cold sensation, a burning sensation, or a numbing sensation as you use ice; stop immediately if the cold becomes unbearable for them.

TIP:
▶ Ice baths are great to prevent swelling after an injury, athletic event, or workout, but they should be done right away (within 24 hours at the latest). If it's been more than a few hours, soak in a warm tub with Epsom salts to restore your electrolyte balance and soothe tired, achy muscles.

COLD COMPRESSES

1. Dip a towel or washcloth in ice water or freeze a wet washcloth for a short period of time.
2. Lay the cloth on inflamed areas to end your partner's massage.

ICE CUBE MASSAGE

1. Freeze a small paper cup full of water.
2. Peel away the top edge of the paper cup.
3. Hold the remaining paper and use the smooth surface of the ice to end your partner's massage.
4. It will melt as you use it. When it melts too much to hold, grab another one.

LOTIONS AND OILS THAT COOL DOWN

1. Spray or smooth a small amount of cooling lotion or oil on your partner's sore or painful area to end your partner's massage.
2. No need to rub it in.
3. If you touched the lotion or oil, don't touch your eyes afterward!

GETTING READY

Before you begin the massage, prepare yourself with proper grooming and a consistent warm-up routine using the following tips.

Groom. Dress the part of a massage therapist. Clip your nails short (most of the white part should be cut off, but don't go too far). Remove your jewelry (even wedding rings), tie back your hair, and use a sweatband across your forehead (to prevent dripping sweat onto your partner). You may also want to tuck a towel around your neck to wipe sweat off your hands and face during the massage. Wear clothes that allow you to move and lunge comfortably, and add a holster around your waist to hold your lotion bottle if there is not a convenient place in the room to keep your bottle. Most important, take a shower and use deodorant before the massage (no natural aromatherapy here, please).

Warm up. Before you start your massage, do the following stretches to warm up your body and mind.

- **Head rolls:** Tip your chin to your chest. Lightly swing your head from side to side. In a rolling motion, allow first one ear, then the other to roll toward the shoulder on the same side, keeping the chin tilted downward. Come to a stop and lift the chin.
- **Shoulder rolls:** Roll the shoulders first backward, then forward several times. With your arms extended to your sides, circle your arms forward, then backward several times. Come to a stop and lower the arms.
- **Spine roll:** Tuck your chin to your chest and roll your body forward and down slowly, with your arms extended toward your toes. Hold the forward fold, then roll back up slowly.
- **Breathwork and grounding exercise:** Close your eyes and take a few deep

breaths. Take a moment to ground yourself (see page 33) with a visualization or by setting your intention for the massage. When you are ready, open your eyes and gently place your hands on your partner to begin the massage.

Test your body in the space: Ensure that you have the proper body mechanics to fit the surface you've chosen for your massage (more information on page 45 in chapter 2):

- **Table, bed, or couch:** Try a standing or kneeling lunge toward your partner.
- **Floor:** Try a kneeling lunge or kneeling (hips on heels), facing your partner.
- **Chair:** Try a standing lunge facing your partner.

Read their body. Finally, evaluate your partner's body mechanics using the next section.

Massage Checklist

✓ Communication, trust, and consent from you and your partner

✓ Clear boundaries and expectations for the massage

✓ Discussion about contraindications and pressure scale

✓ Clean space with plenty of room for your movement

✓ Table, couch, bed, chair, or floor (with padding)

✓ Linens (sheets, blanket, towels)

✓ Bolster, pillow, or towel

✓ Lotion or oil (with holster)

✓ Music player

✓ Scented candle or essential oil diffuser

✓ Lights dimmed

✓ Temperature set around 73 to 77 degrees Fahrenheit

✓ Sweatband and towel for you

✓ Grounding visualization

READING THEIR BODY

Before you begin, ask your partner to stand in front of you, close their eyes, and shake things out. You can learn a lot by looking at their posture and the way they hold their body. For each of the following questions, the first half is "neutral," and the second half indicates a need for massage to release tight muscles.

Neck: Look at your partner's head position. Is their nose pointing forward, or is it turned to one side? Is the top of their head pointing upward, or is it tilted to one side?

Shoulders: Are the shoulders even, or is one shoulder higher than the other?

Arms: Are the thumbs pointing forward, or are they rotated toward or away from the body? Are the elbows relatively straight, or do they look bent?

Hips: Find their hip bones (sticking out on the front of the body). Is one higher than the other?

Legs: Do the toes point forward, or are they rotated to either side? Are the toes lined up, or is one foot forward? Are the legs relatively straight, or do they appear bent at the knee?

Find the bone on the front of the knees (the **patella**). Are they even, or is one patella higher than the other? Is your partner's weight evenly distributed in both feet, or are they leaning more to one side?

Side view of body: Is the chin parallel to the floor, or is it tilted toward the floor or ceiling? Are the following parts in line with each other, or is one out of line: ear holes over shoulders over hips over ankles?

Skin: Is the skin relatively the same color across the body, or does it have patches of different colors? Are there varicose veins or bruises? Is the skin dry, or are there open wounds or oozing patches? Is there bleeding anywhere? Check in with your partner about any areas of caution. (For more information, refer to Contraindications on page 6.)

Note any areas where the body part is turned or tilted away from neutral, and during your massage, work the same side where you noticed the issue. After the massage, ask your partner to stand in front of you and shake it out again, and see the results of your massage in the areas where you worked.

PART 2

Healing Techniques

The following chapters offer a range of healing techniques for different areas of the body. Chapters 4 to 8 cover individual regions of the body and start with a basic sequence that you can use to warm up the area before moving on to specific techniques. These five basic sequences can also be combined into a full-body massage, which you can use to warm up before you address the full-body ailments in chapter 9. Many sections include acupressure points to relieve symptoms of that ailment. See Acupressure Points (page 166) for a diagram of all the acupressure points used in this book.

Start with the Basics

Find your partner's ailment and just do the basic sequence at the beginning of the chapter, which includes rocking and shaking, gliding, and kneading for that area. You can do one or all of these basic techniques and provide a great massage. You can also start with any of the other techniques labeled "Basic Massage," such as acupressure and stretching.

Move on to Advanced Techniques

As you get used to doing massage, you can add in more focused, deeper massage techniques, which are labeled "Advanced Massage." Make sure you use warming moves from the basic sequence (like gliding or kneading) first. Each advanced massage section will tell you the best places to apply the friction and trigger point therapy techniques. Refer to the Fundamental Techniques section in chapter 2 (page 23) for how to do those techniques.

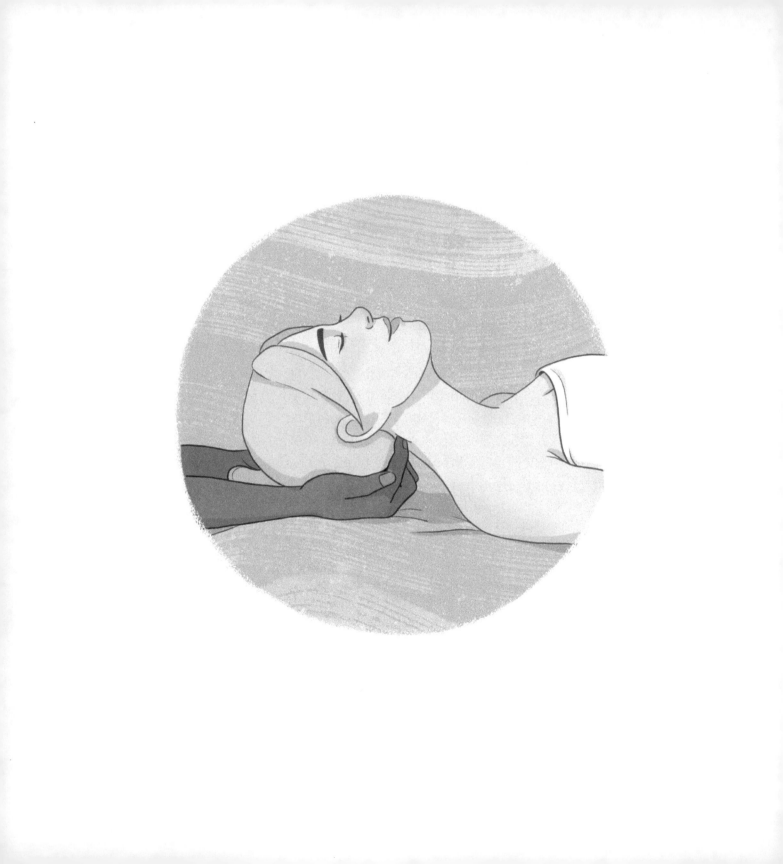

CHAPTER 4

Head, Neck, and Chest

Got a headache or a crick in your neck? You're not alone. Handheld technology, stress, and anxiety in our daily grind causes poor posture, headaches, migraines, neck pain and tension, jaw clenching, and eyestrain. Using our smartphones, we curve forward, shortening the muscles in the chest, increasing the weight of the head, and pulling on the neck and head muscles, leading to chronic head and neck pain. This chapter provides a basic sequence plus basic and advanced massage techniques and tips to relieve pain from the following common ailments in our head, neck, and chest.

HEAD, NECK, AND CHEST SEQUENCE

Gliding (light to medium pressure, 1 to 3)

1. With your partner unclothed and face down, bring the sheet down to uncover their neck. Add lotion to your hands and rub them together to warm the lotion.
2. At your partner's side, place your hands palms down on their neck. Press your hands down lightly, allowing your hands to follow the natural contours of their neck.
3. From your same position, form a C with your hands. Wrap the C around the back of their neck, your thumbs next to each other. Use both hands to slide the C along their neck, one hand at a time, in opposite directions.
4. Continue to glide your hands along your partner's neck with flowing strokes and slow, light pressure, alternating from the top of the neck down to the base of the neck and back up. Repeat until their neck starts to feel soft and warm, adding more lotion as needed.
5. Move to your partner's other side and repeat the C stroke.

Kneading (light to medium pressure, 1 to 3)

1. From the top of your partner's head, use one hand to hold the base of their head, and wrap your other hand around the back of the neck. Use your lunge to press your thumb and fingers into the neck and slide your hand down to the bottom of the neck, repeating and increasing the pressure if needed.
2. Switch hands and repeat.

TIP:
▶ If your partner's head is turned to one side, have them turn it so the other side is facing up when you switch hands.

3. Press the tips of your fingers into their head and press inward, making small circles with each of your fingertips and one large circle with each of your hands.

For the following techniques, have your partner bring their arms out from under the sheet and rest them next to their body outside the sheet. This will hold the sheet in place and give you room to massage their upper chest and neck above the edge of the sheet and hold the sheet in place.

Gliding (light to medium pressure, 1 to 3)

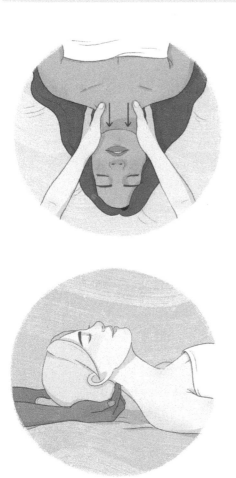

1. With your partner unclothed and face up, add lotion to your hands and rub them together to warm the lotion.
2. Standing at the top of your partner's head, place your hands palms down on the tops of their shoulders. Press your hands down lightly, allowing your hands to move down their arms and follow the natural contours of their shoulders and upper arms, down to their elbows and back up. Repeat a few times.
3. With your fingers under their neck at the base of the neck, lightly press your fingers into the muscles on either side of the spine. Sit back into your lunge and lift the neck slightly with your fingers, sliding your fingers up the neck to the base of their head. Repeat a few times.
4. Hook your fingers into the base of their skull and sit back into your lunge, using your weight to gently pull their head toward you. Hold for a few seconds, then gently release.
5. Use both of your hands to gently lift their head and turn it to their right side. Keep your right hand under their head and cup your left hand

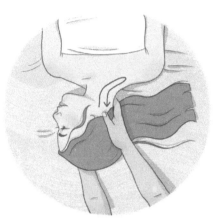

around the top of their neck in a C shape. Use your lunge to gently press your thumb and fingers into their neck and glide down to the shoulder and back up to the base of the head. Repeat a few times on the right side, feeling for different muscles under your fingers each time.

6. Switch their head to the left side and repeat Step 5.

7. Bring their head back to center with their nose pointing upward. Glide your hands from their shoulders down to their elbows and back up again.

8. Place your hands just under your partner's collarbone with your fingers pointing toward each other. Press your hands down lightly, gliding your fingers out toward their shoulders. When you reach their shoulders, turn your hands so your fingers point toward their feet, and glide your hands down their arms, then up the back of their arms and up to the back of their neck. Repeat a few times.

Kneading (light to medium pressure, 1 to 3)

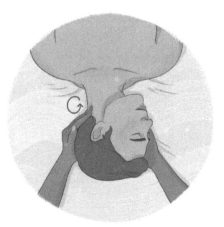

1. Use both of your hands to gently lift your partner's head and turn it to their right side. Gently press your fingers on your left hand into the muscles on the left side of your partner's neck, starting at the base of the head. Firmly and quickly move the fingers down to the base of the neck, making small circles. Repeat a few times, again looking for different muscles under your fingers each time.

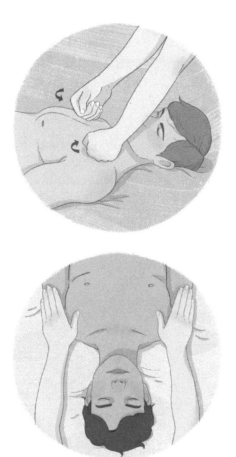

2. Switch their head to the left side and repeat Step 1.
3. Make your hands into soft fists. Press your knuckles and the long bones of your fingers into their muscles just underneath their collarbone (which you may know as the "pecs," short for **pectoralis major**). Glide your soft fists from the center out to their shoulders on both sides. Repeat a few times.
4. Place your palms on the fronts of their shoulders and press their shoulders down into the table, opening the front of their chest.

NECK PAIN

In our culture of chronic stress, neck pain plagues most of us, particularly as we become more dependent on handheld technology. Tilting your head forward to look at your smartphone drastically increases the weight of your head on your neck, resulting in neck pain as your muscles compensate and tense to hold up your head. Your neck muscles weaken over time due to poor posture (when walking, standing, or sitting), misuse, sleeping in awkward positions, carrying heavy bags, whiplash from car accidents, excessive computer use, and many other situations.

Massage can help by relieving stiffness, improving blood flow through arteries that supply blood to parts of the brain, increasing brain functions like concentration and memory, and preventing dizziness, fatigue, headaches, insomnia, and panic attacks caused by neck pain.

> **TIP:**
> ▶ Gentle stretching throughout the day can help with daily neck pain. Try bringing your chin to your chest to stretch the back of the neck, tilting your ear to your shoulder to stretch the side of the neck, and pressing your forearms into a doorway (elbows at shoulder height) to stretch the upper chest muscles. Hold each stretch for a few seconds, then gently release. Repeat as needed throughout the day.

Basic Massage

1. Do the Head, Neck, and Chest sequence (page 60).
2. Use a hot towel or hot stones to warm your partner's neck as you work through the sequence.

Basic Massage: Stretching

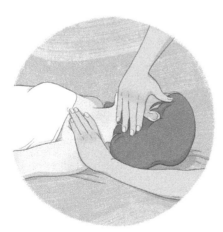

1. With your partner's head turned to the right side, use your right hand to hold the base of their head as your left hand cups their neck and glides down from top to bottom. Hold the stretch at the base of the neck for a few seconds, then gently release. Return their head to the center, then turn it to the left side and repeat.
2. Keep your partner's nose pointing upward, then gently lift their head and move it to the right side, so their ear

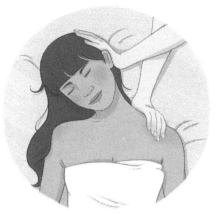

is closer to their shoulder. Place your right hand on their left shoulder at the base of their neck and your left hand on their head just behind their ear. Gently press your hands away from each other to provide a stretch for the side of their neck. Hold the stretch for a few seconds, then gently release. Return their head to the center, then move it so their left ear is closer to their left shoulder and repeat.

Basic Massage: Acupressure (light pressure, 1 to 2)

1. Hold acupressure point GB20, the point just below the base of the head on either side of the neck, about two finger-widths away from the spine. This point reduces stress, calms the mind, improves breathing, and helps with headaches, as well as neck and jaw pain. It also helps with insomnia, fatigue, and general irritability.
2. Hold GB21, the point where your neck meets your shoulder. You can either press down into it or gently pinch the spot using your fingers and thumb. Avoid this point if your partner is pregnant, as it can increase blood pressure. This point relieves headaches and muscle tension in the neck.
3. Hold SI15, the point that is two finger-widths down the back from where the neck and shoulder meet. This point is useful for relieving pain from wear and tear on the bones and cartilage in the neck region, as well as shoulder and neck pain.
4. Hold LI4, the point on the back of the hand in the webbing where the thumb and index finger meet. Avoid this point if your partner is pregnant, as it can induce labor. This point is known as "The Great Eliminator," because it relieves pain of all kinds, including hand, wrist, neck, and back pain. It also boosts the immune system, improves waste elimination, and relieves constipation and symptoms of depression.

Advanced Massage: Friction (medium to firm pressure, 2 to 4)

Warm up your partner's muscles using one or more of the basic massage techniques before moving on to friction.

1. Find the thick muscle along the side of your partner's neck, just to one side of their spine.
2. Use the friction technique (page 26) to release the taut band of muscle in their neck.

TIP:
▶ If your partner's head is turned to the side, use less pressure to protect their neck.

Advanced Massage: Trigger Point Therapy (medium to firm pressure, 2 to 4)

Warm up your partner's muscles using one or more of the basic massage techniques before moving on to trigger point therapy.

1. Find spots on your partner's neck that cause pain (or that send pain to another area of the body) when you press them. This sensation indicates a trigger point in the area.
2. Use the trigger point therapy technique (page 27) on the following areas in your partner's neck that cause or refer pain:

   • The big muscle on the front of their neck (the **sternocleidomastoid**).

   • The small muscles on the side of their neck (including the **scalenes**).

   • The muscles at the base of their head (**suboccipitals**).

   • The muscle that comes down from the top of their neck to their shoulders (the **trapezius**, or "traps").

HEADACHES AND MIGRAINES

Over 45 million Americans suffer from chronic headaches, including tension headaches and migraines. As with neck pain, headaches often result from our culture of chronic stress combined with our recent dependence on handheld technology.

Tension headaches include pain at the temples, as well as eye, jaw, and head pain, and referred pain and muscle spasms in the neck, shoulders, and arms. They can be caused by dehydration, hormonal and chemical changes, muscle spasms, misalignment in the neck, stress and anxiety, and jaw issues.

Migraines are severe headaches that may last for several days. In addition to blinding head pain, you may feel nauseous, throw up, or be sensitive to light and sound. They can be caused by poor regulation of blood sugar, environmental allergens, food sensitivities, stress and sleep issues, nerve and circulation issues, misalignment of the neck, and hormonal and chemical changes.

Massage can help tension headaches and migraines by easing muscle tension, releasing tight muscles in the head, neck, and shoulders, and improving nerve function and circulation. When more oxygen is available for the brain and blood vessels, pain decreases. Massage also switches the body into "rest-and-digest" mode, relieving the anxiety and stress that contribute to headaches.

TIPS:

▶ If you suffer from chronic headaches, use a headache journal. Migraine sufferers often need to journal their food and activity daily to determine their triggers, and carefully monitor their food and water intake, stress levels, and sleep quality.

▶ **Essential oils:** To improve headache pain relief, add your own blend of pain-relieving essential oils to your massage lotion or use a diffuser. Try wintergreen or birch, peppermint, eucalyptus, helichrysum, lavender, chamomile, or cypress. (See page 48 for a safety note on essential oils.)

Basic Massage

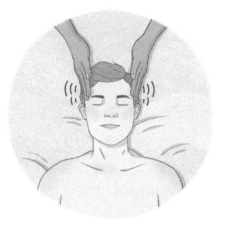

1. Do the Head, Neck, and Chest sequence (page 60).
2. Use a hot towel or hot stones to warm your partner's neck. Place the heat under their neck as you work through the sequence, moving it as necessary.
3. Standing at your partner's head, place your fingers at your partner's temples. Press firmly and make small circles.
4. Continue to make small, firm circles as you move your hands toward the table, massaging the muscle above your partner's ears (the **temporalis**).
5. Spread your fingers apart and press your fingertips into your partner's head, moving their skin and muscles over their skull as you make bigger circles all over the head.
6. Hook your fingers into the base of their head and sit back into your lunge, using your weight to gently pull their head toward you. Lift your hands so their head rises off the table. Allow their head to slowly tilt back over your hands, keeping your fingers hooked into the base of their head. Gently release when their head fully lets go and slowly falls into your hands. Repeat as needed.

Basic Massage: Stretching

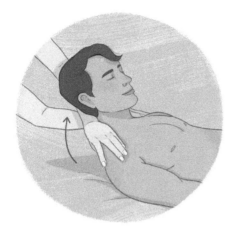

Cross your arms, hands palm-side down, and slide your hands under your partner's head with one hand on each of your partner's shoulders. Cradle their head in your crossed arms and lift, holding their shoulders down for a stretch at the back of the neck.

Basic Massage: Acupressure (light pressure, 1 to 2)

1. Hold the "third eye" point between your partner's eyebrows and just above bridge of their nose. This spot is useful for headaches and earaches.
2. Hold the point at the top of each ear (where the ear bends when you fold it in half). This point is effective for earaches, migraines, and tension headaches.
3. Hold the point where the ear cartilage sticks out, just above the ear hole. This is called the **daith**, and it is so effective for migraine relief that migraine sufferers often get this spot pierced so they have permanent pain relief.

Advanced Massage: Trigger Point Therapy (medium to firm pressure, 2 to 4)

Warm up your partner's muscles using one or more of the basic massage techniques before moving on to trigger point therapy.

1. Find spots on your partner's neck and shoulders that cause pain (or that send pain to another area of the body) when you press them. This sensation indicates a trigger point in the area.

2. Since these spots are on top of the shoulders, you need to use a different hand position to put effective pressure on them. Place your palms together and slide your fingers around the spot, so your palms stay together and one hand is above and one hand is below that spot. You can also grip it between your thumb and index finger, or press into it with supported fingers or supported thumb.

3. Use the trigger point therapy technique (page 27) to release the following areas if they cause or refer pain:

   - The spot where their neck meets their shoulder on one side. This is a hot spot for trigger points in the trapezius muscle.

   - Follow the edge of the trapezius muscle down and out to the shoulder and find the spot where that thick muscle attaches to the bone in the shoulder.

SINUS PRESSURE

Your sinuses are hollow spaces in your skull. You have four pairs of them—**frontal sinus**, in the center of your forehead above each eye; **maxillary sinus**, on either side of your nose below the cheekbones; and **sphenoid sinus** and **ethmoid sinus**, behind your nose. These empty spaces humidify and filter your air, lighten your skull, and enhance your voice. Healthy sinuses have a thin layer of mucus and lots of empty space. When they become inflamed, they produce excess mucus, which causes your congestion, pressure, and pain.

Sinus pressure can be caused by cold, flu, or allergies, as well as structural issues, like uneven nostrils or extra tissue in the nose (called **polyps**). If you suffer from repeated bouts of sinus pressure, you are dealing with chronic sinusitis.

Massage can help by promoting drainage from the sinuses and easing congestion.

TIPS:

▶ Try using a neti pot or other bottle to do nasal irrigation. This is a technique which pushes saltwater into one nostril through all the sinuses and out the other nostril, thinning and clearing excess mucus. There are many affordable kits at your local pharmacy. **Safety note!** Always use distilled or boiled water! Never use tap water, as it may cause bacterial infection.

▶ **Essential oils:** To enhance the feeling of openness, add your own blend of inspiring essential oils to your massage lotion or use a diffuser. Try wintergreen or birch, peppermint, eucalyptus, or cypress. You can also set up a basin of steaming water, put a few drops of oil into the basin, and have your partner breathe in the steam to decrease congestion and open their airways. (See safety note on page 48.)

Basic Massage

1. Do the Head, Neck, and Chest sequence (page 60).
2. Use a warm compress (hot towel or hot stone) on your partner's forehead, cheeks, and over their nose to warm the area. Use a lower temperature here, as the face is more sensitive.

Basic Massage: Frontal Sinus

1. Place your fingers on either side of your partner's forehead, just above the eyebrows.
2. Massage slowly in a circular motion, working your way toward the temples.
3. Lightly tap from the center of your partner's forehead outward, toward the temples.
4. Place your fingers on the inner tips of their eyebrows, pressing lightly into a little notch you will feel in that location. Hold for 1 to 2 minutes.

Basic Massage: Maxillary Sinus

1. Place your fingers on both sides of your partner's nose, in the hollow where the nose and cheek meet.
2. Massage this area in a circular motion for about 30 seconds.
3. Lightly tap this area for another 30 seconds.

Basic Massage: Nose Sinuses

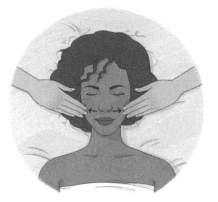

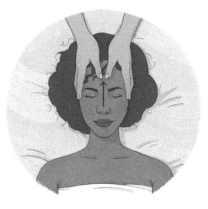

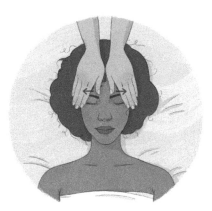

1. Place your fingers on the bridge of your partner's nose. Hold firm pressure toward the center of the nose for about 15 seconds.
2. Next, stroke down along the side of your partner's nose. Repeat slow downward strokes for about 30 seconds.
3. Stroke down to the sides of your partner's nostrils, press in, and pull up toward the forehead, hooking the fingertips under the cheekbones. Hold for a few seconds, then release.
4. With your fingers at your partner's temples, place your thumbs on the bridge of their nose and slide them upward.
5. Place your thumbs at the center of the forehead and firmly stroke outward, toward the temples.

Basic Massage: Acupressure (light pressure, 1 to 2)

1. Hold the "third eye" point between your partner's eyebrows and just above bridge of their nose. This spot is useful for headaches and earaches.
2. Hold LI20, the point at the base on either side of the nostrils where the cheekbone meets the upper jaw. Hook your fingers into the base of the cheekbones and pull up toward the forehead, opening the nostrils.
3. Hold TH17, the point just behind your partner's earlobe. This point is effective for ears that feel stuffed, tinnitus (ringing in the ears), and migraines.

EYESTRAIN

Eyestrain is another common problem in our society, particularly due to our prolonged exposure to computer screens and electronic devices. When our eyes get tired, the eye muscles stop working properly and the surface of the eyes get too dry. When looking at a screen for a long period of time, the eye muscles lose their ability to contract, and focus becomes blurry.

Eyestrain causes fatigue; blurred vision; dizziness; headaches; difficulty focusing; dry, red, and irritated eyes; neck and shoulder strain; eye twitching; and changes in vision.

Massage can help by relaxing the muscles around your eye, increasing circulation to the area and stimulating tear glands to prevent dryness.

> **TIPS:**
> ▶ Start your day standing in front of a sunny window with your eyes closed, allowing sunlight to warm your eyelids. Sunlight helps the retina release dopamine, which is needed for healthy eye development.
>
> ▶ Use a warm or cold compress to relieve eyestrain by dipping a cloth into clean water and placing the cloth over your eyes for a few minutes while you lie down and relax. For puffiness, wrap the cloth around a few ice cubes and place it over your eyes.

- To relax tired eyes, rub your hands together until they are warm, then place your cupped palms over your closed eyes. Ensure that no light enters your eyes and settle into the dark for a few minutes. Reenter the light slowly, opening your eyes inside your hands before removing them away from your face.

- When working in front of a screen, follow the 20-20-20 rule. Every 20 minutes, gaze at least 20 feet into the distance for at least 20 seconds.

Basic Massage

1. Do the Head, Neck, and Chest sequence (page 60).
2. Use a hot towel or hot stones to warm your partner's face. Use a lower temperature for warming the face, as this area of the body is more sensitive.
3. Gently massage your partner's forehead and the ridges along the top and bottom of your partner's eyes with your fingertips.
4. Lightly hook your fingers under the eyebrow ridges and hold pressure there.
5. Lightly press your fingers into the bones under your partner's eyes, moving from the bridge of their nose out to their temples with small circles. Be sure to hold pressure at the inner and outer corners of their eyes.
6. Spread your fingers apart and massage the sides of your partner's head above the ears, pressing firmly to move the skin and muscle over their bone.
7. Firmly massage the top and back of the head with your fingertips, as if you were washing your partner's hair.

Basic Massage: Acupressure (light pressure, 1 to 2)

1. Hold UB2, the point where the top of the nose meets the eyebrow. The point is in a little notch that is tender to the touch. This point is wonderful for relieving headaches, eyestrain, and other eye issues.
2. Hold UB1, the point on either side of the bridge of the nose where your glasses normally rest. This point helps with headaches, red, itchy, or painful eyes, allergies, and other eye problems.

3. Hold ST1, the point on the bone under the center of the eye. This point is effective for red eyes, nearsightedness, night blindness, allergies, and excessive tears.

JAW TIGHTNESS

Jaw tightness is caused by clenching or grinding your teeth, usually a habit brought on by stress or anxiety. You may be dealing with TMJ, shorthand for **temporomandibular joint syndrome**. Symptoms of TMJ syndrome include jaw pain, clicking, ear pain and ringing, dizziness, tension headaches, and toothaches. Dentists were the first health-care professionals to recognize the healing power of massage, since they would pull out aching teeth only to find their patients still having pain in the empty socket!

Jaw muscles connect to the jawbone (**mandible**), the cheekbone, and the side of the head (**temporal bone**). The large muscle at the corner where the jawbone meets the cheekbone and head is called the masseter. The muscle on the side of the head is called the **temporalis**, and it comes under the cheekbone and attaches underneath the **masseter**. Massaging the muscles in this area will reduce your TMJ symptoms. Be careful with the pressure just in front of the ear and behind the edge of the jaw. There is a delicate tip of bone there, and very firm pressure could damage it.

> TIPS:
>
> ▶ Talk to your dentist about grinding or clenching, and ask about being fitted for a mouthguard.
>
> ▶ Keep your tongue between your teeth during the day to prevent daytime clenching.
>
> ▶ Add daily stress-relieving techniques (see page 160) to reduce TMJ symptoms caused by stress or anxiety.
>
> ▶ Use the techniques to relieve headaches and neck pain, which often lead to jaw tightness.

Basic Massage

1. Do the Head, Neck, and Chest sequence (page 60).
2. Use a hot towel or hot stones to warm your partner's face. Use a lower temperature for warming the face, as this area of the body is more sensitive.
3. Explore the cheek and jaw area with your fingertips, using light to medium pressure to locate the areas with achy tension. Glide along any knotted fibers you feel in the masseter. Use your supported thumb or fingertips to work quick, firm friction circles into the knots, working along and across the fibers to create heat.

Basic Massage: Stretching (firm pressure, 3 to 4)

1. Firmly press your fingertips into the masseter with your partner's mouth slightly open.
2. Have your partner open their mouth as slowly as they can as you glide your fingertips upward, pinning their jaw muscles against their cheekbones.
3. Hold with your partner's mouth open to stretch the masseter.

Basic Massage: Acupressure (light pressure, 1 to 2)

1. Hold TH17, the point just behind your partner's earlobe. This point is effective for jaw pain, ears that feel stuffed, tinnitus (ringing in the ears), and migraines.
2. Hold SI19, in the notch in front of your partner's ear (by the curled part of the ear). This point is useful for jaw pain, tinnitus, ear infections, earaches, and migraines.
3. Hold GB20, the point just below the base of the head on either side of the neck, about two finger-widths away from the spine. This point reduces stress, calms the mind, improves breathing, and helps with headaches, as well as neck and jaw pain. It also helps with insomnia, fatigue, and general irritability.

Advanced Massage: Trigger Point Therapy (medium to deep pressure, 2 to 4)

1. Check if any spots in your partner's jaw or head muscles cause pain (or that send pain to another area of the body) when you press them. This sensation indicates a trigger point in the area.
2. Use the trigger point therapy technique (page 27) on each spot in your partner's jaw or head muscles that causes or refers pain.

FACE TENSION

Facial tension often accompanies headaches, migraines, jaw issues, and sinus pressure. Stress and anxiety also cause facial tension, which includes tingling, redness, lip damage, and headaches.

Massage can help by increasing circulation to the face, relieving tension, reducing puffiness, toning the muscles of the face, and increasing collagen production. Massage has the added benefits of preventing wrinkles and brightening your skin tone.

TIPS:

▶ Try some facial exercises daily to stretch and tone your face muscles. You can try holding a wide smile; allowing your jaw to soften and open with your tongue on the roof of your mouth; raising your eyebrows as high as possible; closing your eyes as tightly as possible; and scrunching your nose. Hold each pose for several seconds, release, and repeat.

▶ When massaging the face, always stroke upward, toward the top of the head. This direction encourages lifting the muscles and helps prevent sagging and wrinkles.

▶ You can use a forward fold from standing to invert the head below the heart and get a rush of blood to your face. This is a great way to warm up before face massage or face exercises.

Basic Massage

1. Do the Head, Neck, and Chest sequence (page 60).
2. Use a hot towel or hot stones to warm your partner's face. Use a lower temperature here, as the face is more sensitive.
3. Place your fingers at your partner's temples and massage firmly with small circles, moving upward along their hairline.
4. Massage their forehead with small circles from their eyebrows up to their hairline.
5. Place your fingers on either side of the bridge of your partner's nose and press inward as you glide up to the forehead.
6. Glide your fingers across your partner's cheeks, from nose to ear.
7. Using your thumb and index finger, lightly pinch their jawline from chin to ear.
8. Massage their jawline from chin to ear with small circles.
9. Starting on the forehead, lightly tap your fingertips across their forehead, cheeks, and jawline.

EARACHE

Earaches have many causes, including jaw issues, ear infections, referred pain, allergic reactions, water trapped in the ear, and changes in altitude. Ear infections often accompany sinus pressure, sore throats, and headaches. Pain is often due to inflammation and fluid in the **eustachian tube**, which connects the ear to the nose and throat. This tube is meant to drain the middle ear into the throat and prevent the mucus in your runny nose from entering your ear canal.

> TIP:
> ▶ Warm and cold compresses can help with earache pain. Try both and see which one relieves your pain—every earache is different. You can also try garlic oil drops in the ear, which is said to reduce inflammation and relieve earaches.

Basic Massage

Do the Head, Neck, and Chest sequence (page 60).

Basic Massage: Eustachian Tube Massage (light pressure, 1 to 2)

1. Place your supported fingers behind your partner's earlobes, in the groove between the earlobes and the jaw.
2. Tilt their head slightly to one side.
3. Using steady pressure, slide your fingers downward until you meet their collarbone.
4. Repeat a few times, then do it with the head tilted slightly to the other side.

Basic Massage: Acupressure (light pressure, 1 to 2)

1. Hold TH17, the point just behind your partner's earlobe. This point is effective for ears that feel stuffed, tinnitus (ringing in the ears), and migraines.
2. Hold SI19, in the notch in front of your partner's ear (by the curled part of the ear). This point is useful for tinnitus, ear infections, earaches, and migraines.
3. Hold the point at the top of the ear (where the ear bends when you fold it in half). This point is effective for earaches, migraines, and tension headaches.

SCALP RELIEF

Your head has several muscles under the scalp, including temporalis (over the ears), **frontalis** (on the forehead), and the **occipitals** and **suboccipitals** (at the base of the skull). There is also a large sheet of fascia covering the top of your head. Muscles and fascia of the head can be tight and tense for many reasons, including stress, anxiety, insomnia, chronic headaches or sinus pressure, or neck and shoulder tension. A sore, tense, or itchy scalp can be distracting and painful.

Scalp massage has been used for centuries to influence the body's energy, balance, and function, particularly in the Ayurvedic tradition. A warm oil massage conditions the scalp, strengthens the roots of the hair, nourishes the hair, and relaxes the muscles in the scalp and neck area. Scalp massage also stimulates circulation, reduces muscle tension, promotes hair growth, improves lymphatic drainage, relieves migraines and headaches, and lowers blood pressure and heart rate. It relaxes the body and mind, boosts memory and energy levels, and relieves symptoms of anxiety, depression, and insomnia.

TIPS:

▶ Scalp massage helps with a dry or itchy scalp when paired with tea tree oil, thanks to its antiseptic properties. Massage the oil into your partner's scalp and hair roots and leave it on overnight for maximum benefit.

▶ Choose your strokes carefully, depending on your partner's needs. Slow movements are best for relaxation. Vigorous movements increase energy and circulation in the head and neck.

Basic Massage

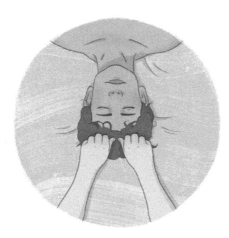

1. Do the Head, Neck, and Chest sequence (page 60).
2. Using dry hands, spread your fingers and press your fingertips into your partner's scalp, gliding your fingers around their entire head. Turn their head to each side and glide your fingers along the muscles on the sides of their head.
3. Press your fingertips more firmly into their scalp and massage all areas of their head with small circles.
4. Use your thumbs and knuckles to make small circles all over your partner's head, warming up their scalp and their muscles and fascia underneath.

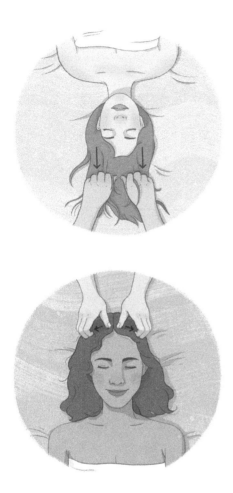

5. Stretch the sides of their scalp by pressing supported fingers or thumbs into the sides of your partner's head above the ear. Press firmly and slide your hands up to the top of the head, holding for several seconds. Gently release.

6. With your thumbs at the center of the top of your partner's head and your fingertips curled, use your thumbs to press into the scalp and move toward the ears. Work your hands back from the hairline to the top of the head, repeatedly pressing the thumbs outward from the center.

7. With your partner's permission, gather up their hair in one big bunch at the top of their head and gently pull it toward you, lifting the scalp off the skull. For short hair, gently grip a handful of hair and squeeze your hand into a fist, lifting the scalp. This move is an excellent stretch for the scalp and feels lovely when done properly. It should not be painful!

8. Warm some massage oil between your hands by rubbing them together.

9. Use your fingertips to work the oil into your partner's scalp, moving their hair as needed. Work the oil into their entire scalp, from their hairline in front to their hairline in back and around the ears.

10. Your partner can leave the oil on for a while (even overnight, covering their pillow with a thick towel). Wash it out with a gentle shampoo.

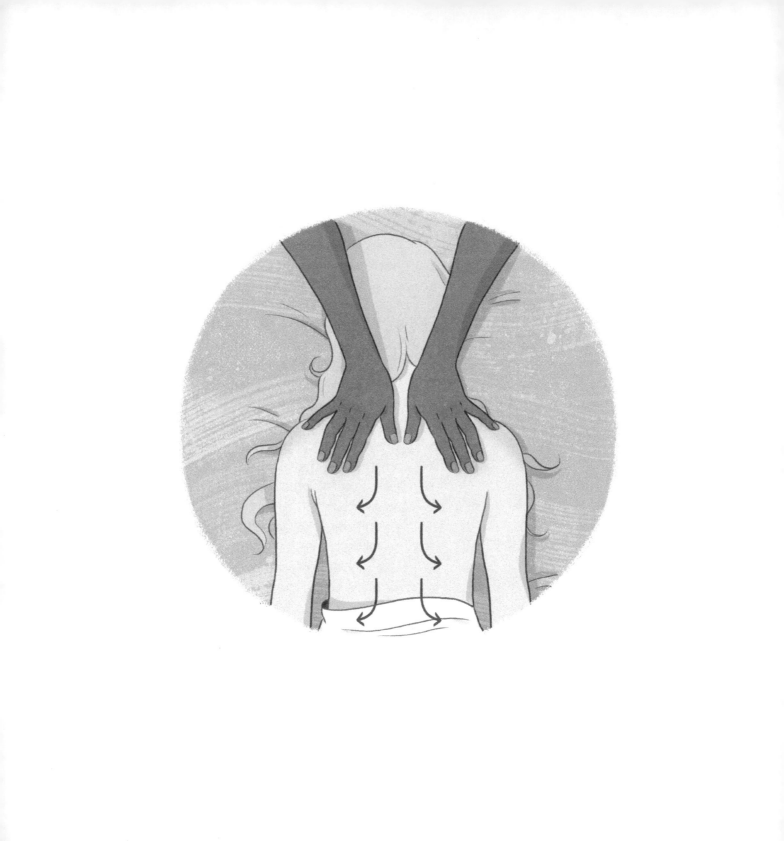

CHAPTER 5

Back and Shoulders

In our culture of chronic stress, sometimes it feels like we carry the weight of the world on our shoulders. Like with head and neck pain, smartphones, stress, and daily activities cause poor posture, back and shoulder tension, and lower-back pain that become chronic as they go untreated. This chapter provides a basic sequence plus basic and advanced massage techniques and tips to relieve pain from the following common ailments in our back and shoulders.

BACK AND SHOULDERS SEQUENCE

Basic Massage: Rocking and Shaking (light pressure, 1 to 2)

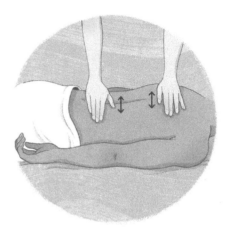

1. With your partner lying face down, start with one hand at the base of their neck and your other hand at the base of their spine. Lightly press down and move your hands away and toward you at a pace that moves the whole spine. Find your partner's rhythm and continue rocking for several minutes. As your partner relaxes, the rhythm may slow down.
2. Turn your partner over, so they are lying face up. Use a soft fist at their shoulder and another soft fist at their hip to rock your partner's spine back and forth.

Basic Massage: Gliding (light to medium pressure, 1 to 3)

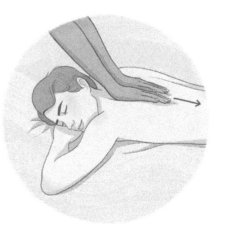

1. With your partner lying unclothed and face down, bring the sheet down to uncover their back. Add lotion to your hands and rub them together to warm the lotion.
2. Standing at the top of your partner's head, place your palms down on their back. Press your hands down, allowing them to follow the natural contours of their body.
3. Glide your hands along your partner's back with long, flowing strokes and slow, light

pressure from the tops of their shoulders down to their lower back. Repeat until their back starts to turn pink and feel soft and warm, adding more lotion as needed.

4. Next, add more lotion and glide your hands from the base of their neck out to their shoulders and upper arms, repeating until their shoulders start to turn pink and feel soft and warm.

Basic Massage: Kneading (light to medium pressure, 1 to 3)

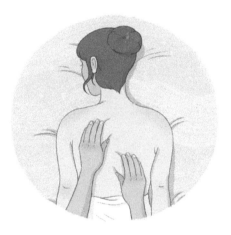

1. Once you've warmed their back and shoulders with gliding, press your hands and fingers more firmly into their back and shoulders with these kneading techniques.
2. From the top of your partner's head, form a C with each hand and use the C to gently lift the skin and muscle on your partner's back, sliding your hands from the outside of their back in toward their spine. Repeat the move from the top of their shoulders down to their lower back.
3. From your partner's side, reach across their body to their opposite shoulder where their neck and shoulder meet. Loosely hook your fingertips underneath their muscle and lean back, stretching it. Using one hand at a time, hook your fingers under their neck-shoulder junction and slide your hand back toward you, replacing it with your other hand, which also slides back toward you. Repeat until the area loosens.
4. Switch sides and repeat on their other shoulder.

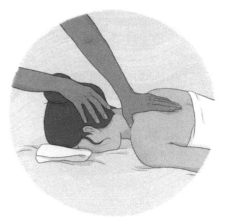

5. From the top of your partner's head, use one hand to hold the base of their head, and hook your other thumb into the place where their shoulder meets their neck. Use your lunge to press your thumb into this space and slide your hand down and out to their shoulder.

6. Switch hands and repeat on their other shoulder.

Advanced Massage: Friction (medium to firm pressure, 2 to 4)

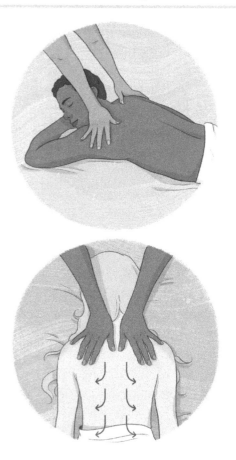

1. From the top of your partner's head, press your thumbs into the muscles on either side of their spine and alternate pressure between your hands as you glide your hands down their back.

2. Repeat, this time moving your thumbs outward at the same time toward your partner's sides instead of alternating pressure between your hands.

3. Still from the head of the table, but now working on just one side, press your palms and fingertips of each hand, one at a time, into their muscles on one side of their spine, replacing one hand with the other in a shingling effect all the way from their shoulder to their lower back. Repeat on their other side.

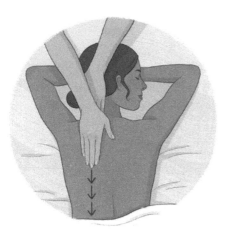

4. Moving to your partner's side, press your thumbs and knuckles into the muscles on the same side of their spine, starting at their lower back and going up to the base of their neck. Move to the other side of your partner and repeat.

5. Still on your partner's side, find the edges of their shoulder blade on one side (it is triangle-shaped, with the point at the bottom and a flat edge at the top). Feel for the thick muscle on top of their shoulder blade. Press the pads of your stacked fingers or supported thumbs into that muscle perpendicularly (so your pressure is directed across the shoulder blade, toward the spine).

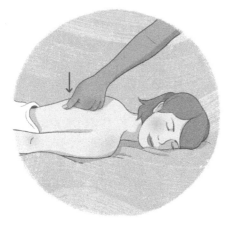

6. Firmly and quickly press your fingers across the muscle on your partner's shoulder blade and across the muscles between their shoulder blade and spine.

7. Move back to the top of their shoulder blade on the same side. This time, keep your fingers pointing toward their feet (instead of across the shoulder blade) as you press into the muscle on their shoulder blade. Make circles with the pads of your fingers with small, deep strokes from the top of the shoulder blade to the pointed bottom.

8. Repeat on the muscles between their shoulder blade and spine.

9. Switch to your partner's other side and repeat on their other shoulder blade.

BACK PAIN

Back pain is a huge problem for people today. 80 percent of Americans will have at least one episode of lower-back pain during their lifetime, and back pain costs employers over 264 million lost workdays per year. It is the sixth-most expensive condition treated in the United States every year. 8 percent of American adults (16 million people) currently suffer from chronic back pain that limits their abilities in some way.

Back pain encompasses a wide range of issues, from pain due to poor posture to nerve impingement causing pain in the back, neck, and the rest of the body. The spine runs from the base of the head down to the tailbone inside the **pelvis**. It is made up of seven **cervical** vertebrae, 12 **thoracic** vertebrae, five **lumbar** vertebrae, along with the **sacrum**, tailbone, and **discs** between the vertebrae. The spine contains the **spinal cord**, which branches off into **nerves** that exit between the vertebrae and run out to send signals to the body and limbs. The curves in the spine make it sturdy and flexible, allowing a full range of movement (bending and twisting) as well as strength and stability. There are many joints within the spine itself, along with **ligaments** and **muscles** that connect to and move the spine.

Such intricate structure means there are many opportunities for dysfunction. Falling, lifting heavy objects, overuse, straining a muscle, spraining a ligament, poor posture, sedentary living, accidents, injuries, long periods of sitting, and normal wear and tear all contribute to back pain. Acute back pain, lasting for only a few days or weeks, comes on suddenly after an accident or injury. Chronic back pain lasts for more than three months, and may be gradual, constant, occasional, or related to movement or position (including sleep). Chronic pain tends to include stiffness and reduced mobility in the back and neck. Issues causing back pain also include disc issues (bulging, herniated, or degenerative discs, specifically), arthritis, osteoporosis, and structural issues (like one leg being longer than the other, or one side of the pelvis being shorter than the other).

Since the nerves originate in the back, issues in the back may radiate to the corresponding parts of the body where the nerves go. Upper-back pain can radiate to the arms, chest, and abdomen, while lower-back pain radiates to the glutes, legs, and feet. There may also be tingling, numbness, or weakness in the corresponding areas, which indicates some nerve impingement or damage.

Massage can help by relieving tension, restoring circulation and improving range of motion for the back and neck.

Basic Massage

1. Do the Back and Shoulders sequence (page 84).
2. **Vibration:** Using stacked hands, press your palms into the muscle on top of your partner's shoulder blade and stiffen your arms to vibrate the area. Pause as needed—it's tough on your body! Repeat on the muscles between their shoulder blade and spine, and work both sides.

Basic Massage: Acupressure (light pressure, 1 to 2)

1. Hold KI27, the fleshy point just below where your collarbone meets your breastbone. This point relieves throat, chest, and back pain and encourages deep breathing.
2. Hold TH3, the point on the back of the hand between the pinky and ring finger tendons, about one finger-width down from the knuckle. This point relieves tension, including neck and upper back pain caused by tension or stress.
3. Hold GV14, the point on the spine at the center of the upper back, just above the top edge of the shoulder blades. This point is effective for relieving stiffness and pain in the neck and upper back.

Advanced Massage: Trigger Point Therapy (medium to firm pressure, 2 to 4)

Warm up your partner's muscles using one or more of the basic massage techniques before moving on to trigger point therapy.

1. Find spots on your partner's upper back that cause pain (or that send pain to another area of the body) when you press it. This sensation lets you know there is a trigger point in that spot.

2. Use the trigger point therapy technique (page 27) on the following areas on your partner's upper back that cause or refer pain:

   - The muscles on top of their shoulder blade (the **supraspinatus** and **infraspinatus**).

   - The muscles between their shoulder blade and spine (the **rhomboids**).

   - The muscle that covers the back in a diamond shape from the base of the head out to the shoulders and down to the spine at the middle of the back (the trapezius).

   - The group of muscles that tuck into both sides of the spine (the **erector spinae group**, which feels like thick ropes right next to the spiny bumps on the back).

   - The muscle that covers the mid-back like a wing and attaches to the top of the upper arm (the **latissimus dorsi**, which you may know as the "lats").

   - You can also bring your partner's arm overhead and massage the muscles on the ribs underneath the shoulder blade (the **serratus posterior superior**) and the muscle tucked inside the front of the shoulder blade (the **subscapularis**).

LOWER-BACK PAIN

Lower-back pain is common in today's sedentary Western culture. In a study covering two years' time, nearly 29 percent of American adults reported having lower-back pain in the past three months, and over 35 percent of people who reported lower-back pain had pain radiating into their leg as well (see Sciatica, page 121).

The most common cause of lower-back pain is a sprained ligament or strained muscle, including tears (which you may call a pulled muscle or "throwing your back out"). Back sprains and strains can occur in a variety of circumstances, including lifting heavy objects, twisting or leaning over while lifting, repeated bending or crouching, falling, poor posture, running on uneven pavement, sitting for long periods of time, sports injuries, and car accidents.

Being overweight and out of shape, severe coughing, poor sleep, and high levels of stress can also trigger chronic lower-back pain. Chronic lower-back pain may also result from bulging or ruptured discs between the vertebrae, issues with the joints between the vertebrae or with the joints between the spine and the pelvis, narrowing of the spinal cord canal (**stenosis**), wear and tear on vertebral joints (**osteoarthritis**), and other structural and hereditary issues.

There is a square muscle that attaches to the ribs, spine, and pelvis and causes much of our lower-back pain (the **quadratus lumborum**). It is responsible for helping lean to one side and, more often, hiking the hip on one side to hold something heavy (like holding a baby on your hip).

Massage can help by relaxing the back and neck muscles, releasing adhesions caused during the healing process, addressing deeper muscle tightness in the lower back, pelvis, and abdomen, and improving symptoms of stress, anxiety, and insomnia.

TIPS:

▶ Stretch your lower back daily to increase your flexibility and range of motion. Lie on the floor, bring your knees to your chest, and rock from side to side to loosen your lower back. Put your left foot flat on the floor and bring your right knee to your chest, then cross your right ankle over your left knee and lift your left foot off the floor, hugging your left leg into your chest. Repeat on the other side to fully stretch the lower back.

▶ A kneeling lunge will soften the front of the hip and release tight hip and abdominal muscles, which contribute to lower-back pain, particularly when there is poor posture or limited core strength.

Basic Massage

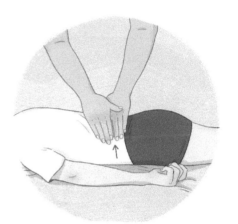

1. Do the Back and Shoulders sequence (page 84).
2. Move to one side of your partner. Press the heel of one hand into their lower back, and reach across with your other hand and pull the opposite side toward you, so you are lifting their lower back slightly between your hands. Rock their lower back between your hands as both hands glide toward the spine, releasing before they touch the spine.
3. Switch hands and repeat.
4. Still from the side, reach across your partner with both hands and loosely hook your fingertips under the opposite side. Lean back, lifting their lower back and stretching the lower-back muscles you've hooked into. Using one hand at a time, hook your fingers under and slide the hand back toward you, replacing it with the other hand, which also slides back toward you. Repeat until the area loosens.
5. Switch sides and repeat Steps 2 to 4 on the other side of their lower back.

Basic Massage: Stretching

1. From your partner's right side, cross your arms and hook your right hand into their ribs and your left hand into their hipbone. Use your lunge to press your hands apart and stretch their side, particularly the **quadratus lumborum**.
2. From your partner's head, stack your palms over their tailbone and press down toward their feet to stretch their lower back.

Basic Massage: Acupressure (light pressure, 1 to 2)

1. Hold UB23, the point on the back midway between the ribs and the hipbone, one finger-width away from the spine. This point relieves lower-back tension, kidney-related issues, sexual issues, earaches, coughs, and asthma.

2. Hold UB47, the point on the back that is three finger-widths away from the spine and three finger-widths down from the corner of the shoulder blade. This point relieves tension in the quadratus lumborum muscles, helps with vomiting, diarrhea, and breathing problems, and reduces symptoms of depression and anxiety.

3. Hold UB54, the point on the back of the leg in the middle of the crease of the knee. This point relieves stiffness and lower-back pain caused by disc and nerve issues (including **sciatica**), knee pain and stiffness, leg pain, muscle spasms, skin problems, and issues with overheating.

Advanced Massage: Trigger Point Therapy (medium to firm pressure, 2 to 4)

Warm up your partner's muscles using one or more of the basic massage techniques before moving on to trigger point therapy.

1. Starting on one side of the lower back, find the edges of the **quadratus lumborum** by locating the top of your partner's hip bone (the **pelvis**), their lower-back (**lumbar**) spine, and the bottom of their ribs.

2. First, find spots on your partner's lower back that cause pain (or that send pain to another area of their body). This sensation tells you there is a trigger point in that spot.

3. Use the trigger point therapy technique (page 27) on the following areas in your partner's lower back that cause or refer pain:

   • Where their spine meets the bottom of their ribs.

   • Where their hipbone meets their spine.

- On the edge of this muscle toward the side of your partner's body where it doesn't attach to any bones. You will likely feel a thick, dense band of muscle. Making a C with your hands, hook your thumbs under that band and press up and in until you find another tender spot.

- On your partner's tailbone (the low-lower back).

- On your partner's upper glutes, just below the edges of the hipbones.

SHOULDER TENSION

Shoulder pain and tension have many causes, from stress and anxiety to rotator cuff injuries and frozen shoulder. The shoulder is a ball-and-socket joint, so it is highly mobile and can perform many different movements. The rotator cuff is actually a group of four muscles, including supraspinatus, infraspinatus, **teres minor**, and subscapularis, that keep the end (or **head**) of the upper arm bone (the **humerus**) in its socket. The most common injuries in the shoulder happen when the head does not stay centered in the socket, including tears, frozen shoulder, bone-on-muscle impingement, swelling and inflammation, and cartilage and other tissue dysfunction.

Neck, shoulder, and arm pain also result from **thoracic outlet syndrome**, which is diagnosed when the nerves that run from the neck to the arm are compressed in one or more outlets

TIPS:

▶ Sometimes doctors diagnose patients with carpal tunnel syndrome without checking for thoracic outlet syndrome; since they have similar symptoms, be sure your doctor tests for and can treat both conditions. You may even have both conditions. Massage can help by releasing adhesions in shoulder muscles, increasing mobility and circulation, decreasing shoulder pain, and relieving symptoms of stress and anxiety associated with pain.

▶ If part of your partner's shoulder is inflamed (swollen, soft, and squishy, and possibly red or warm to the touch), you can still massage areas that are not inflamed. Use cool compresses or ice on the inflamed areas, and heat on the tense or stiff (but not inflamed) areas.

between muscles and bone. The nerves for the arm are bundled together in the **brachial plexus**, which runs through two small neck muscles (**anterior** and **middle scalenes**), then under the collarbone and a small muscle called the **subclavius** above the first rib, then under **pectoralis minor**, a small strap-like muscle that forms the front edge of your armpit. If any of these muscles are tight, they will compress the arm nerves, causing pain, tingling, numbness, and weakness in the forearm, wrist, hand, and fingers.

Basic Massage

1. Do the Back and Shoulders sequence (page 84).
2. Do the Head, Neck, and Chest sequence (page 60).

Basic Massage: Stretching

Cross your arms, hands palm-side down, and slide your hands under your partner's head with one hand on each of your partner's shoulders. Cradle their head in your crossed arms and lift, holding their shoulders down for a stretch at the back of the neck.

Basic Massage: Acupressure (light pressure, 1 to 2)

1. Hold GB20, the point just below the base of the head on either side of the neck, about two finger-widths away from the spine. This point reduces stress, calms the mind, improves breathing, and helps with headaches, as well as neck and jaw pain. It also helps with insomnia, fatigue, and general irritability.
2. Hold GB21, the point where your neck meets your shoulder. You can either press down into it or gently pinch the spot using your fingers and thumb. Avoid this point if your partner is pregnant, as it can increase blood pressure. This point relieves headache and muscle tension in the neck.
3. Hold LI16, the point in the depression at the top of the shoulder where the trapezius meets the shoulder blade and the collarbone. This point is useful for addressing shoulder issues, increasing circulation, and improving balance and attention.

Advanced Massage: Trigger Point Therapy (medium to firm pressure, 2 to 4)

Warm up your partner's muscles using one or more of the basic massage techniques before moving on to trigger point therapy.

1. Find spots on your partner's shoulder that cause pain (or that send pain to another area of the body) when you press it.
2. Use the trigger point therapy technique (page 27) on the following areas in your partner's neck that cause or refer pain:

   - The muscles on top of their shoulder blade (the supraspinatus and infraspinatus).

   - The muscles between their shoulder blade and spine (the rhomboids).

   - The muscles on the outside edge of the shoulder blade that attach to the upper arm (**teres major** and teres minor).

   - The muscle that runs from the upper corner of the shoulder blade to the neck (the **levator scapula**).

   - The muscle that covers the back in a diamond shape from the base of the head out to the shoulders and down to the spine at the middle of the back (the trapezius).

   - The thick round cap of muscle that covers the tops of the shoulders (the **deltoids**, or "delts").

   - The long muscles on the upper arms (**triceps brachii** on the back, and **biceps brachii** on the front).

   - You can also bring your partner's arm overhead (hanging off the table) and massage the muscles on the ribs underneath the shoulder blade (the serratus posterior superior) and the muscle tucked inside the front of the shoulder blade (the subscapularis).

Advanced Massage: Trigger Point Therapy: Ribs
Under the Shoulder Blade (medium to firm pressure, 2 to 4)

1. To massage the muscles on the ribs underneath the shoulder blade (**the serratus posterior superior**), bring your partner's arm up and around so it hangs off the table or lies in front of them. This move brings their shoulder blade off the ribs and exposes the muscle, which I like to call "the secret knot."

   - **Secret knot tip:** When someone tells me they have had a lot of massages and have never felt relief for their shoulder pain, I always massage this muscle. This muscle works to keep the shoulder blade over the ribs, but in our culture of constantly having our arms forward for typing and handheld devices, it is frequently overworked and overstretched.

2. Find the edge of your partner's shoulder blade (much farther out to their side now) and sink your supported fingers or thumbs into their muscle underneath. Glide toward the spine and repeat many times until the area is pink and warm, working up and down the edge of their shoulder blade and across to their spine.

3. Use the trigger point therapy technique (page 27) on this area for any spot that causes or refers pain for your partner.

Advanced Massage: Trigger Point Therapy: Underside
of the Shoulder Blade (medium to firm pressure, 2 to 4)

1. There are two ways to massage the muscle tucked inside the front of your partner's shoulder blade (the **subscapularis**). This muscle helps keep their shoulder blade on their ribs, and it is similarly overworked and overstretched. It is often bulky and can cause the tip of their shoulder blade to stick out from their back. With your partner's arm still forward, bring your hands palm-side up to the outer edge of their shoulder blade.

2. Press your fingertips up into their muscle under the bony edge of their shoulder blade (on the side that is normally against the ribs), making small circles if possible.

3. Use the trigger point therapy technique on this area for any spot that causes or refers pain for your partner.

4. Now bring your partner's hand back around and bend their arm at their elbow, placing their hand at their lower back (if possible).
5. Find the upper tip of their shoulder blade that now sticks up at the base of the neck where it meets their shoulder.
6. Hook your fingers under that tip into the muscle along the bony edge and sink back into your lunge.
7. Use the trigger point therapy technique on this area for any spot that causes or refers pain for your partner.

Advanced Massage: Trigger Point Therapy: The "Traps"
(medium to firm pressure, 2 to 4)

1. To massage trigger points in the trapezius muscle that cause shoulder pain and tension, find the spot where their neck meets their shoulder on one side. This is a hot spot for trigger points in the trapezius muscle. You can also follow the edge of the trapezius muscle down and out to the shoulder and find the spot where that thick muscle attaches to the bone in the shoulder.
2. Use the trigger point therapy technique (page 27) on both of these areas if they cause or refer pain for your partner.

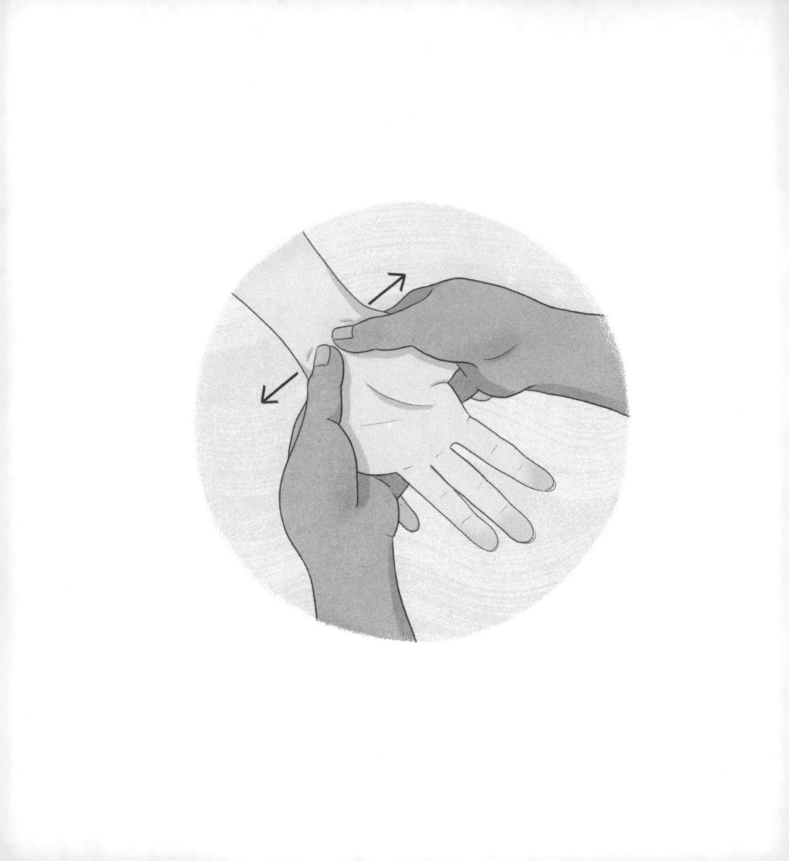

CHAPTER 6

Arms and Hands

With computers and office work, we use our arms and hands more than ever before. Daily use and maintenance of machines, cars, computers, and handheld technology cause poor posture, repetitive use injuries, and pain in our forearms, wrists, and hands. This chapter provides a basic sequence plus basic and advanced massage techniques and tips to relieve pain from the following common ailments in our arms and hands.

ARMS AND HANDS SEQUENCE

Basic Massage: Rocking and Shaking (light pressure, 1 to 2)

1. With your partner lying face up, start with one hand in a soft fist at their shoulder and your other hand pressing lightly at their wrist. Lightly press down and move your hands away from and then toward you at a pace that moves their whole arm. You can also use one hand on either side of their arm to rock it back and forth between your hands. Find your partner's rhythm and continue rocking for several minutes. As your partner relaxes, the rhythm may slow down.
2. Bring your partner's arm out from under the sheet and let the sheet fall, resting their arm on top of the sheet.
3. Bend your partner's arm at the elbow and hold their forearm between your palms, moving your hands up and down it as if you're starting a campfire.
4. Wrap your hands loosely around their wrist and shake their hand back and forth.

Basic Massage: Gliding (light to medium pressure, 1 to 3)

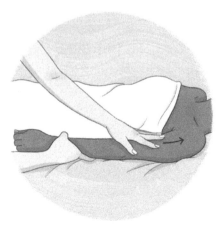

1. With your partner unclothed and face up, move the sheet to uncover their arm.
2. Add lotion to your hands and rub them together to warm the lotion.
3. At your partner's side, place your hands palm-side down on their arm. Press your hands down, allowing your hands to follow the natural contours of their arm.
4. Glide your hands along your partner's arm with long, flowing strokes and slow, light pressure from the shoulder down to the hand. Repeat until the arm starts to feel soft and warm, adding more lotion as needed.

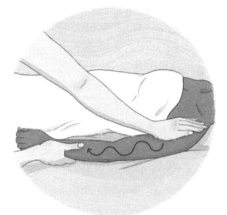

5. Hold just below your partner's wrist with one hand and glide the other hand upward, holding the arm in place.

6. Place your hand palm-side down on your partner's shoulder and hold their upper arm with your other hand in a C shape. Sit back in your lunge and use your thumb to trace a curvy line as you glide your hand down their upper arm and forearm.

Basic Massage: Kneading (light to medium pressure, 1 to 3)

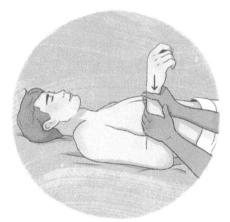

1. Still at their side, form a C with your hands and wrap the C around their upper arm, thumbs next to each other. Use both hands to slide the C along the upper arm, one hand at a time, in opposite directions (one hand up their arm, the other down their arm). Move your hands to their forearm and repeat.

2. Hold your partner's hand palm-side down in both of your hands, pressing your fingers into their palm and pulling them apart. Repeat a few times.

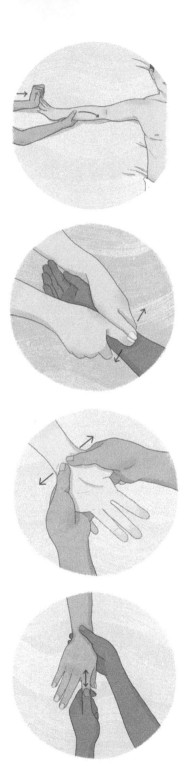

3. Bend your partner's arm at the elbow and hold their hand in both your hands again, this time with your thumbs on their palm. Use your thumbs to knead their palm, holding their hand steady with your fingers.

4. With their elbow still bent, wrap your hands around their forearm and glide your hands down to their elbow.

5. Bring your partner's arm out to the side, holding their fingertips with one hand and gently pressing them toward your partner's shoulder. Cup their forearm with a C shape with your other hand and glide up to their elbow, stretching their forearm muscles.

6. Hold your partner's hand with both of your hands, placing your thumbs on the center of their wrist. Press firmly and spread your thumbs apart to the edges of the wrist. Knead their palm with your thumbs.

7. Still holding their hand with both of your hands, put one of your pinkies between their ring and pinky fingers and the other pinky between their thumb and index finger. Use your thumbs again to open the wrist as you spread them toward the edges. Knead their palm with your thumbs to increase the relief.

8. Turn their hand over. Hold their wrist with one hand and gently rub and pull each finger one at a time.

FOREARM PAIN AND CARPAL TUNNEL SYNDROME

Forearm pain has many causes, including hereditary conditions, injuries (like fractures and sprains), compressed nerves (like carpal tunnel syndrome and thoracic outlet syndrome), overuse, and wear and tear on the elbow and wrist joints (like **tendinitis** and **tendinopathy**). Nerves may be compressed by poor posture, muscle tension due to overuse (like sports with throwing, catching, and swinging, as well as contact sports), and scar tissue from injuries. Tendon inflammation (tendinitis) and pain (tendinopathy) occur near the elbow and wrist where the tendons connect muscles to bones. They usually cause pain, swelling, weakness, and difficulty moving the arm and hand.

The carpal tunnel is on the palm side of the wrist. It is created by nine tendons and one nerve crossed over by a wide ligament band. Carpal tunnel syndrome occurs when the tendons are thickened or inflamed by overuse or injury, compressing the nerve and causing pain, tingling, numbness, and weakness in the hand and fingers.

> **TIPS:**
>
> ▶ Carpal tunnel syndrome is often misdiagnosed. Thoracic outlet syndrome also causes pain, tingling, numbness, and weakness in the arm, hand, and fingers due to compression of arm nerves in the neck and shoulder. When you seek medical advice, be sure your medical provider assesses for and can treat both conditions. You should receive massage in your neck and shoulders in addition to your hand and forearm for more complete pain relief.
>
> ▶ If you work with your arms forward, stretch your chest muscles frequently by clasping your hands behind your back or bringing your arms up with the elbows bent ("cactus arms") and leaning into a doorway with your forearms on the doorjamb. Do arm circles and shoulder shrugs often to loosen tight chest and shoulder muscles.
>
> ▶ Take frequent breaks when working or exercising to ensure that your wrists are not in the same position for more than 30 minutes. Keep your forearms level with the keyboard while typing. Use your hands evenly, taking turns with tasks using your right and left hands. Use proper posture when sitting and standing.
>
> ▶ Wearing a wrist splint during repetitive motions like typing and while sleeping can ensure proper alignment and relieve the pressure on the nerve at your wrist. You can buy comfortable wrist splints with cushy pillows inside them for sleeping.

Carpal tunnel syndrome may be caused by long-term repetitive motions. Some of these motions include computer use, assembly line work, cycling, yoga, weight lifting, or mechanic and plumbing work. Carpal tunnel syndrome is hereditary (small tunnels), so you may be more likely to develop this syndrome if either of your parents have dealt with it. Diseases like diabetes and **rheumatoid arthritis** can also contribute to carpal tunnel syndrome symptoms.

Massage therapy can help by decreasing tension in the hand and forearm, which relieves inflammation, pain, and numbness in the area. Massage will also release adhesions, scar tissue, and trigger points in the hand and forearm muscles that result from inflammation and contribute to the symptoms, restoring full range of motion to the wrist.

Basic Massage

1. Do the Head, Neck, and Chest sequence (page 60).
2. Do the Back and Shoulders sequence (page 84).
3. Do the Arms and Hands sequence (page 102).

Basic Massage: Stretching

1. Bend your partner's arm at the elbow so their palm is facing you.
2. Cup your hand in a C shape and hold your partner's wrist. Cup your other hand in a C and wrap it around their palm (with your thumb on their palm between their thumb and index finger).
3. Bend their hand back at their wrist as you press your other thumb into their wrist, providing a wrist and palm stretch.
4. Repeat, this time gliding your hand down their forearm as you bend their hand back, providing a forearm stretch.
5. Bring their arm down with the palm facing the table. Cupping your hands into C shapes again, hold their wrist with one hand and their hand with your other hand, this time with your fingers on their palm and your thumb on the back of their hand.

6. Press your thumb into their wrist as you bend their hand forward this time, providing a stretch for the wrist and the back of the hand.
7. Repeat, this time gliding your hand up their forearm as you bend their hand forward, providing a forearm stretch.

Basic Massage: Acupressure (light pressure, 1 to 2)

Hold PC6, the point that is three finger-widths down from the crease of the wrist on the inner forearm, in the center between the two thickest tendons. This point relieves pain and fullness in the chest, anxiety, depression, insomnia, nausea, motion sickness, and wrist pain, and, particularly, the symptoms of carpal tunnel syndrome.

Advanced Massage: Friction (medium to firm pressure, 2 to 4)

Warm up your partner's muscles using one or more of the basic massage techniques before moving on to friction.

1. Place your partner's hand on the table, palm down.
2. Find a taut band of muscle tension that resists your pressure in the forearm, and use the friction technique (page 26) to release it.
3. Once you feel the muscle release (the band softening), use gliding strokes to "warm out" and relax their muscle before moving on.
4. Repeat the friction technique on all areas of muscle tension in the forearm that you can find.
5. Turn your partner's arm over and repeat Steps 2 to 4 on the palm side of the forearm.

Advanced Massage: Trigger Point Therapy (medium to firm pressure, 2 to 4)

Warm up your partner's muscles using one or more of the basic massage techniques before moving on to trigger point therapy.

1. Find spots on your partner's forearm that cause pain (or that send pain to another area of the body) when you press it. This sensation indicates that a trigger point is present.
2. Use the trigger point therapy technique (page 27) on the following areas in your partner's neck that cause or refer pain:

   - With your partner's palm down, the muscles near the elbow, about halfway down the forearm, and on the thumb side and pinky side of the wrist. These are all **extensor** muscles that move the hand and fingers.

   - With your partner's palm up, the muscles near the elbow, about halfway down the forearm, and on the thumb side and pinky side of the wrist. These are all **flexor** muscles that move the hand and fingers, plus the **pronator teres**, which turns the hand palm up or palm down.

   - **Note:** On this side of the forearm, there is no need to do massage past halfway down to the wrist, as the muscles all become tendons after that point, and trigger point therapy is effective only on muscles, not tendons.

WRIST AND HAND PAIN

Wrist and hand pain can make your life difficult, limiting your everyday activities, like dressing, bathing, preparing food, and opening doors. This pain can be caused by conditions like sprains, strains, chronic arthritis (worn-down cartilage between two bones resulting in painful bone-on-bone contact), osteoarthritis, rheumatoid arthritis, diabetes, pregnancy, obesity, and **trigger finger** (a stiff tendon that causes your finger to catch when it is straightened). Tennis elbow (**lateral epicondylitis**) and golfer's elbow (**medial epicondylitis**) are inflammatory conditions in tendons of the elbow that also cause wrist and hand pain. For pain caused by carpal tunnel syndrome, see the previous section.

Repetitive hand tasks like typing, painting, handwriting, playing musical instruments or sports, and using tools can also cause pain, cramping, and tension in your hands and wrists. There are several conditions that are usually diagnosed in worker's compensation cases due to the wear and tear on the tendons, muscles, and nerves caused by continuous use over an extended period. These are known as RSI (**repetitive strain injury**), CTD (**cumulative trauma disorder**), RMI (**repetitive motion injury**), and MSD (**musculoskeletal disorder**), and they are used interchangeably. Contributing factors include working with bent wrists or neck, extended arm reach, long periods in a fixed position (particularly in awkward postures), task repetition, excessive pressure on muscles and joints, incorrect lighting levels, and excessive pinch grips while writing.

Massage can help by reducing hand pain, increasing grip strength, and improving mood and sleep. Massage also increases circulation in the hands, which relieves pain and speeds healing after injury. It also hydrates connective tissue, releases adhesions, and softens scar tissue in your hands and fingers, improving your hands' range of motion and flexibility. Friction massage followed by stretching is particularly effective to help relieve pain and tension associated with trigger finger.

TIPS:

▶ For hand and wrist pain, it is important to do forearm massage in addition to wrist and hand massage. Many trigger points in the forearm refer to the hand and wrist, as do many nerve issues in the neck, shoulders, and arms.

▶ Ensure that your desk setup is **ergonomic;** you can do an Internet search for "ergonomic office" and find some tutorials. Some of these will suggest using boxes and stands to adjust your desk, computer, and chair. If you work at a company with more than 50 employees, they are required to have an ergonomic specialist and make reasonable accommodations to set up your workspace ergonomically.

▶ To further decrease pain in tendon issues, massage your partner's sore tendon with ice after doing friction massage and stretching. The ice will prevent additional swelling and speed healing.

▶ If your partner feels numbness or tingling at any time during the massage, stop your pressure immediately; this sensation indicates you are putting pressure on a nerve.

Basic Massage

1. Do the Back and Shoulders sequence (page 84).
2. Do the Arms and Hands sequence (page 102).
3. (Advanced) Do the friction, trigger point therapy, and stretching techniques in the Forearm Pain and Carpal Tunnel Syndrome section (page 105).
4. With your partner's hand palm up, hold their hand with both your hands, placing your thumbs on their palm.
5. Gently massage their palm with your thumbs, starting in the center and working outward.
6. Using your thumbs, firmly massage the fleshy pads on the thumb side and pinky side of your partner's palm.
7. Pinch the edges of the pinky side of their palm firmly between your thumb and index finger knuckle.
8. Holding the base of each finger with your index finger and thumb, massage the base of each finger and the flesh between the fingers with your thumb.
9. Turning your partner's hand palm down, press your thumbs into the grooves between the finger tendons on the back of the hand, making small circles up to the wrist.
10. Pinch the sides of each finger firmly, above and below their knuckle, holding for a few seconds in each spot.
11. Pinch the tips of each finger firmly, holding for a few seconds.

Basic Massage: Acupressure (light pressure, 1 to 2)

1. Hold LI4, the point on the back of the hand in the webbing where the thumb and index finger meet. Avoid this point if your partner is pregnant, as it can induce labor. This point relieves pain of all kinds, including hand, wrist, neck, and back pain.
2. Hold SI3, the point just below the pinky finger where the palm creases when your hand makes a loose fist. This point is useful for neck and back pain, headache, red and painful eyes, and hand pain.
3. Hold pressure in the webbing between each finger, using your thumb and index finger on both sides of your partner's hand. These points are effective for hand pain and osteoarthritis in the hands.

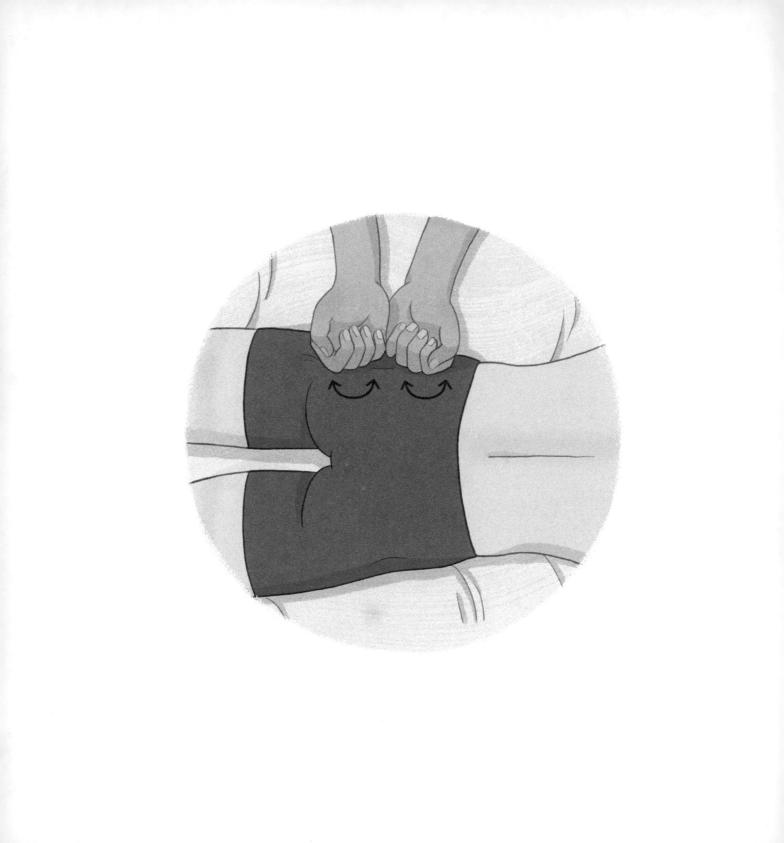

CHAPTER 7

Hips

As we move to a more sedentary lifestyle, particularly with the advent of office and computer work and long work commutes, the muscles in the front of our hips and our buttocks get short, tight, and tense, causing hip and sciatic pain. This chapter provides a basic sequence plus basic and advanced massage techniques and tips to relieve pain from the following common ailments in our hips.

HIPS SEQUENCE

Basic Massage: Rocking and Shaking (light pressure, 1 to 2)

1. With your partner lying face down, start with one hand at the base of their spine and your other hand in a soft fist at the side of their hip. Lightly press your soft fist into their hip away and then toward you at a pace that moves the whole spine. Find your partner's rhythm and continue rocking for several minutes. As your partner relaxes, the rhythm may slow down.
2. Place one hand in a soft fist on your partner's glutes. Raise your partner's lower leg with your other hand at their ankle so the knee is bent at a 90-degree angle.
3. Bring their foot toward and then away from you, rotating the upper leg bone in the hip socket. Press down with your soft fist to stretch and warm the glutes.

Basic Massage: Gliding (light to medium pressure, 1 to 3)

1. With your partner unclothed and lying face down, bring the sheet down to uncover their back. Fold the sheet back to uncover one of their hips. Add lotion to your hands and rub them together to warm the lotion.
2. Standing at your partner's side, place your hands palms down on their lower back and upper hip. Press your hands down, allowing your hands to follow the natural contours of their body.
3. Glide your hands from the side of their back and hip to the center (the spine and tail-bone), all along the lower back and glutes. Repeat, using short, flowing strokes and slow, light pressure until their hip and glutes start to turn pink and feel soft and warm, adding more lotion as needed.

Basic Massage: Kneading (light to medium pressure, 1 to 3)

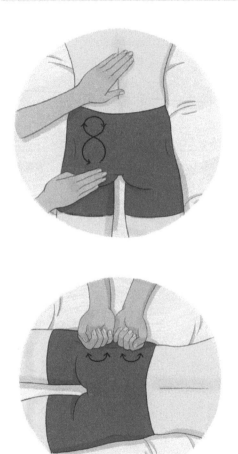

1. Once you've warmed their hip and glutes with gliding, press your hands and fingers more firmly into their hip and glutes with these kneading techniques.
2. From your partner's side, form a C with each hand and use the C to gently lift the skin and muscle on your partner's hip and glutes, sliding your hands from the edge of their body of their back in toward their spine and tailbone. Repeat the move from their hipbone down to the bottom of their glutes, following the contours of the hipbone, tailbone, and sit bone (**ischial tuberosity**, one of the bony points you feel when you sit on the floor, at the bottom of their glutes, where their **hamstrings** connect).
3. Press the heels of your hands into their hip and glutes, flowing smoothly toward the spine and tailbone from the top of the hip to the bottom of the glutes.
4. With one hand on their lower back, use your supported fingers or thumb to make a figure 8 on your partner's glutes.
5. Make soft fists and press your knuckles and long finger bones into your partner's glutes, twisting to soften and move the muscles.

Advanced Massage: Friction (medium to firm pressure, 2 to 4)

Warm up your partner's muscles using one or more of the basic massage techniques before moving on to friction or trigger point therapy.

1. With stacked hands or supported thumbs, find their hipbone and make small friction circles where the muscles meet the bone, massaging from the side of their hip up and over to the tailbone, then down the edge of the tailbone.
2. Repeat the line of small circles where the muscles meet the sit bone at the bottom of the glutes.
3. Find a tough dense tissue between the tailbone and the sit bone, which is a thick ligament that connects the two bones. Make small friction circles and vibrate your fingers with pressure on that ligament to soften it.
4. Find a taut band of muscle tension that resists your pressure in your partner's hip and glutes.
5. Use the friction technique (page 26) to release any taut bands of muscle in their hip and glutes.

Advanced Massage: Trigger Point Therapy (medium to firm pressure, 2 to 4)

1. Find spots on your partner's hip and glutes that cause pain (or that send pain to another area of the body) when you press it. This sensation indicates a trigger point is present.
2. Use the trigger point therapy technique (page 27) on the following areas:

    *   The muscles along the hipbone at the top of the glutes.

    *   The muscles between the top of the leg bone and the tailbone (including the **piriformis**).

    *   The muscles along the tailbone.

    *   The muscles that connect to the top of the sit bone. These are the **gluteus maximus**, **gluteus medius**, and **gluteus minimis** muscles, which are layered on top of each other in the gluteal region.

HIP TIGHTNESS

Hip tightness is generally caused by tension in your hip flexors, which are muscles at the top of the leg connecting the leg bone (**femur**) and the pelvis that allow you to bend at the waist and lift your upper thigh. In our sedentary society, our hip flexors are held in a constantly contracted position and are often shortened by a few inches and are much weaker than they should be, causing pain, tension, and a decreased range of motion in the hip.

Postural and structural issues can also cause hip tightness, including a tipped pelvis, a pelvis or leg bone that is shorter on one side than the other, leaning on one side when standing, or sleeping with one leg up on one side and not supporting the knee with a pillow. Weight lifters, CrossFitters, and other gym enthusiasts regularly lifting and squatting also deal with frequent hip tightness. Trigger points in the glutes cause hip pain as well.

Hip tightness is sometimes mistaken for core weakness, resulting in many sessions of ill-advised crunches and sit-ups following by back pain and more hip tightness. One overlooked muscle in our bodies is the **psoas** muscle, a long, slender strip that runs from either side of the spine in the middle back, down through the pelvis, and to the top of the inner thighbone. This is the only muscle connecting our legs and back, and it is actually the cut of meat that results in filet mignon in a cow. Instead of being tender and soft, however, our chronically shortened psoas is usually dehydrated, dense, and 2 to 3 inches shorter than its proper length.

The psoas is the muscle that contracts when we are afraid, curling us into the fetal position to protect the tender and vital belly, heart, and face. Having the psoas in a constantly shortened position tricks the brain into thinking we are in a chronic state of danger, heightening anxiety and stress in addition to tensing and dehydrating the psoas. The psoas is also a stabilizing muscle for the spine and a sling-like support for the abdominal organs, so trigger points in the psoas muscle show up as back pain, disc problems, sciatica, scoliosis, hip degeneration, knee pain, digestive problems, shortness of breath, and even issues with organ function.

Massage can help tight hips by breaking down scar tissue and adhesions in the hip flexors, releasing trigger points and secreting endorphins to reduce pain, and increasing blood flow to relax their muscles.

▶ Hip pain is often misdiagnosed as pain due to sciatica (irritation of the sciatic nerve running through the glutes and down the leg) or arthritis (worn-down cartilage between two bones, resulting in painful bone-on-bone contact), when muscle tension and trigger points are most likely to blame. Be sure your medical professional considers all alternatives and listens carefully to the location of your pain and the sensations, like numbness and tingling (or not) that accompany it. You can refer to the Sciatica and Arthritis sections (pages 121 and 150) for more information on those conditions.

▶ Upward-Facing Dog pose and kneeling lunges are two great stretches for the fronts of the hips.

Basic Massage

Do the Hips sequence (page 114—you can do just the basic sections, or add on the advanced if you're ready).

Basic Massage: Rocking and Shaking (light pressure, 1 to 2)

With your partner lying face up, place your hands in soft fists at the side of their hip. Lightly press your soft fists into their hip away and then toward you at a pace that moves the whole lower torso. Find your partner's rhythm and continue rocking for several minutes. As your partner relaxes, the rhythm may slow down.

Basic Massage: Gliding (light to medium pressure, 1 to 3)

1. With the sheet still covering them, find their hipbone. Lightly press your fingers down that bone and onto the leg, finding the muscles and ligaments that run from hip to leg. These muscles are the hip flexors.
2. Uncover your partner's hip and tuck the blanket between their legs. Add lotion to your hands and rub them together to warm the lotion.

3. Standing at your partner's side, place your hands palms down on the top of their leg near the knee. Press your hands down, allowing them to follow the natural contours of their body.

4. Glide your hands from their knee up the front of the thigh, using long, flowing strokes and slow, light pressure and ending up with both hands at the side of their hip. Repeat until their leg and the front of their hip start to turn pink and feel soft and warm, adding more lotion as needed.

Basic Massage: Kneading (light to medium pressure, 1 to 3)

1. From your partner's side, form a C with each hand and use the C to gently lift the skin and muscle on your partner's leg and the front of their hip, gliding your hands from the knee up to the hip (one hand moving down the leg, the other moving up the leg).

2. Press the heels of your hands into the sides of their leg, flowing smoothly toward the hip.

3. Make soft fists and press your knuckles and long finger bones into your partner's leg, gliding up the leg to the hip.

Basic Massage: Stretching

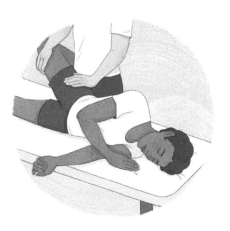

1. Have your partner turn to their opposite side and hold on to the far side of the table.

2. Facing their back, place one hand on their ankle and one hand at their knee.

3. Bend their knee and bring their ankle and knee toward you, turning yourself toward their feet to bring their leg behind them and around your waist.

4. They should feel the stretch in the front of their hip. Hold for at least a minute, then stretch them a little farther, holding again. Release gently by bringing their leg back to their body.

5. Have your partner turn over, so they are lying face down.

6. Place your hand under their ankle. Bending their leg at the knee, bring their ankle to their glutes. To increase the stretch, put your knee on the table under their knee to lift their leg off the table. They should feel the stretch in the front of the hip and all along the **quadriceps** muscles, or "quads."

Advanced Massage: Friction (medium to firm pressure, 2 to 4)

Warm up your partner's muscles using one or more of the basic massage techniques before moving on to friction.

1. Find their hipbone on the front of their hip and slide your fingers just inside the bone, making small friction circles as you glide down along the bone and onto the leg.

2. Find a taut band of muscle tension that resists your pressure in the front of your partner's hip and upper leg.

3. Use the friction technique (page 26) to release any taut bands of muscle in their hip and upper leg.

Advanced Massage: Trigger Point Therapy (medium to firm pressure, 2–4)

Warm up your partner's muscles using one or more of the basic massage techniques before moving on to trigger point therapy.

1. Find spots on your partner's hip and upper leg that cause pain (or that send pain to another area of the body) when you press it. This sensation indicates a trigger point is present.

2. Use the trigger point therapy technique (page 27) on the following areas in your partner's hip and upper leg that cause or refer pain:

   • The muscle along the inside of the hipbone (the **iliacus**).

   • The big muscle on the front of the thigh that crosses from the upper leg to the hipbone (the **rectus femoris**, one of the muscles in the quadriceps group).

- The attachment of the long strap-like muscle on the outer edge of the hip bone (the **sartorius**).

- The small thumb-sized muscle on the outer upper leg (the **tensor fascia latae**, which contracts to tighten the IT band).

Advanced Massage: Psoas Release (medium to firm pressure, 2 to 4)

Warm up your partner's muscles using one or more of the basic massage techniques before moving on to trigger point therapy.

1. To release your partner's psoas, you'll need 20 to 30 minutes to allow your fingers time to settle into your partner's abdomen.
2. Curl your fingers over the hipbone.
3. Allow the weight and warmth of your fingers to sink into the muscle on the hipbone (the **iliacus**). Use your lunge to hold this light pressure for several minutes. You'll notice your fingers sinking deeper into your partner's abdomen.
4. After 15 minutes or so, your fingers will slide far enough down the hipbone and move your partner's organs aside to allow your fingers to settle on their psoas muscle, which will likely feel dense, ropy, thick, and tough.
5. Using stacked fingers, apply a tiny bit more pressure and use the trigger point therapy technique (page 27) on this spot. Your fingers may slide upward along the psoas (toward your partner's head) as you hold pressure.

SCIATICA

Up to 40 percent of adults will experience **sciatic pain** at some point in their lifetime, which is a stabbing, burning, or shooting pain from the lower back that travels down the back of the leg (usually on just one side). True sciatica is a condition in which the sciatic nerve, which runs through the glutes from either side of the lower back, is irritated or compressed at the nerve root in the lower back, causing pain, tingling, numbness, or weakness in the lower back, leg, and foot.

True sciatica can be caused by injuries in car accidents, nerve root irritation by a herniated lumbar disc, a pinched nerve due to a fractured vertebra, degenerative discs or narrowing of the spinal canal (stenosis), and sometimes pregnancy (due to the weight of the uterus on the sciatic nerve). Prolonged sitting can make sciatica worse. The symptoms of true sciatica can be relieved somewhat by massage, but it is difficult to treat and nearly impossible to heal without surgery.

When the sciatic nerve is compressed by muscles in the glutes, you may suffer sciatica-like symptoms, but it is actually **piriformis syndrome** and not true sciatica. Under the muscle layers of the gluteus maximus and gluteus medius, there are six small, deep muscles that help stabilize and rotate the top of the leg bone in the hip socket. In most bodies, the **sciatic nerve** runs under the **piriformis** and over the other five muscles. Tension in these six muscles (and especially the piriformis) can compress the sciatic nerve and cause sciatic pain. In some people, the sciatic nerve runs over the piriformis. In just 5 percent of people, the sciatic nerve runs through the piriformis, which is a debilitating condition usually caught early and corrected by surgery.

Massage can help with piriformis syndrome and true sciatica by loosening and lengthening tight muscles compressing the sciatic nerve, particularly the piriformis, which will restore nerve function and drastically reduce pain. Massage also improves circulation and lymph flow, which boosts the body's ability to heal itself, restores range of motion for the leg and hip, eases symptoms of anxiety and depression connected with chronic sciatica, and even improves sleep.

TIPS:

▶ Sciatica is often misdiagnosed when patients report hip pain, particularly when the pain moves down the leg. However, in addition to piriformis syndrome, several trigger points in the glutes refer pain down the leg, often accompanied by stiffness, a feeling of heaviness in the leg, and a dull ache throughout the leg and glutes (without the stabbing or shooting pain that usually indicates nerve compression). Be sure your medical provider is aware of muscular issues and considers all alternatives before diagnosing you with sciatica.

▶ Stretching during the massage is important, since stretching helps release compression of the nerve by the muscles in the glutes and keeps them lengthened and loose. Add regular hip stretches into your routine for more lasting pain relief.

▶ During flare-ups of sciatic pain, alternate heat and ice on the affected glutes, always starting with heat and ending with ice.

Basic Massage

Do the Hips sequence (page 114, basic and advanced), paying special attention to the muscles between the top of the leg bone and the tailbone (including the piriformis).

Basic Massage: Stretching

1. With your partner lying face up, have them bend their knees and place their feet flat on the table.
2. Grasp the ankle on the leg that has sciatic pain and press their knee to their chest, stretching the glutes.
3. Place that ankle on their other knee in a figure 4 shape. With one hand on the upright thigh under the knee and your other hand on the outside edge of their crossed knee, press their knees and thigh toward their chest, stretching the outer glutes and the piriformis.
4. Release gently and bring their legs back down to the table.

Basic Massage: Acupressure (light pressure, 1 to 2)

1. Hold GB30, the point near the top of the leg bone on the side of the glutes, one-third of the way to the tailbone. This point is effective for weakness, numbness, and pain in the legs, lower-back pain, sciatica, and piriformis syndrome.
2. Hold GB34, the point on the side of the lower leg, about three finger-widths down from the knee just behind the leg bone (**fibula**). This point is useful for numbness and pain in the legs, swelling and pain in the knee, shoulder pain, and joint and ligament issues.

Advanced Massage: Friction (medium to firm pressure, 2 to 4)

Warm up your partner's muscles using one or more of the basic massage techniques before moving on to friction.

1. The piriformis is a long triangle with the flat end at the tailbone and the point at the top end of the leg bone on the lower side of the glutes. After the top layer of glutes have been warmed and loosened, you will be able to feel the thick, tight piriformis between the leg bone and tailbone in the center of the glutes.
2. With your partner lying face down, locate the piriformis muscle.
3. Use the friction technique (page 26) to release tension in the piriformis.

Advanced Massage: Trigger Point Therapy (medium to firm pressure, 2 to 4)

Warm up your partner's muscles using one or more of the basic massage techniques before moving on to trigger point therapy.

1. Find a spot on your partner's piriformis that causes pain (or that sends pain to another area of the body) when you press it. This sensation indicates a trigger point is present.
2. Use the trigger point therapy technique (page 27) to release any trigger points you find in the piriformis.

PMS

Premenstrual syndrome, or PMS, is a combination of physical and emotional symptoms occurring 1 to 2 weeks prior to menstruation due to the change in hormones that create the menstrual cycle. Physical symptoms include headache, acne, tender breasts, bloating, back pain, constipation, and fatigue. Emotional symptoms include irritability, mood swings, and increased symptoms of depression and anxiety. Not all women have these issues during menstruation, but 80 percent report suffering from PMS at some point during their lives. 75 percent of those who deal with symptoms of PMS do not treat their symptoms, and those with the most severe symptoms are the least likely to treat them.

Massage can help by reducing cramping and pain in the abdomen, promoting circulation to help with bloating, and decreasing symptoms of anxiety and depression. Massage can also release trigger points in the upper leg associated with pelvic pain and cramping. Light abdominal massage increases circulation and lymph flow, decreases fluid retention, and calms the nervous system, helping to reduce both physical and emotional symptoms.

> **TIPS:**
> ▶ Before your symptoms begin, cut back on alcohol, caffeine, and soda to reduce bloating. You can also exercise to relieve menstrual cramps and reduce stress, which may help with emotional and physical PMS symptoms. Keep a journal to see when your PMS symptoms are the worst and identify any triggers to avoid before and during your period.
> ▶ **Essential oils:** To further relieve PMS symptoms, add your own blend of soothing essential oils to your massage lotion or use a diffuser. Try clary sage, lavender, bergamot, chamomile, ylang ylang, cedarwood, or geranium. (Do not use clary sage if your partner is pregnant!)

For the following techniques, have your partner lie face up (with a pillowcase or towel on their chest, under the sheet). Add lotion to your hands and rub them together to warm the lotion.

Basic Massage: Gliding (light pressure, 1 to 2)

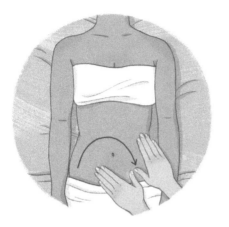

1. Bring the sheet down to uncover your partner's stomach. Face toward your partner's head and place your hands gently on their stomach, framing their belly button with your thumbs.
2. Once your partner is accustomed to your touch, place your hands palm down on the right side of their abdomen, starting with your palms near the right hipbone, and then glide over the belly button to the left hipbone. Repeat gently.

Basic Massage: Kneading (light to medium pressure, 1 to 2)

1. Bring the sheet down to uncover your partner's stomach. Facing your partner, stack your hands over their lower abdomen and lightly press down, vibrating your hands to relax the lower abdominal muscles and the uterus.
2. Still with stacked hands, press the heels of your hands lightly into their stomach and push away from you, then pull back softly toward you with your fingers. Repeat in a fluid paddling motion.
3. Reach across your partner's body with one hand, sliding your fingers under the opposite side of their lower back. Pull your hand back toward yourself, softly raking your fingers across their lower belly. Push the heel of your other hand into your partner's near side, lightly pressing the heel of your hand across their lower belly. Alternate pushing and pulling with your hands to knead the lower abdomen.
4. Uncover your partner's leg and tuck the sheet under their other leg. Bend their leg at the knee and place it down with the sole of their foot on the other leg so that their inner thigh is exposed.

5. Add lotion to your hands and rub them together to warm the lotion.

6. Standing at your partner's side, place your hands palms down on the inside of their leg near the knee. Press your hands down, allowing your hands to follow the natural contours of their body.

7. Glide your hands from your partner's knee up the inside of their thigh, using long, flowing strokes and slow, light pressure and ending up with both hands at the top of their leg. Repeat until their leg starts to turn pink and feels soft and warm, adding more lotion as needed.

Basic Massage: Stretching

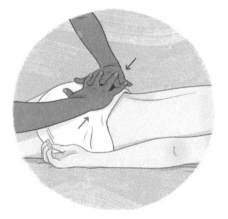

1. Stand at your partner's side, facing their head. Clasp your hands over their tailbone and press the heels of your hands into the sides of their tailbone, lifting as you press.

2. Move to their head and face their feet. Stack your hands over their tailbone and press the heels of your hands down, pushing toward your partner's feet to stretch their lower back.

Basic Massage: Acupressure (light pressure, 1 to 2)

1. Hold CV6, the point that is two finger-widths down from the belly button at the center of the abdomen. This point is helpful for irregular periods, menstrual cramps, and vaginal discharge. It can also relieve gas, irritable bowel syndrome, headache, and general weakness.

2. Hold SP8, the point that is four finger-widths down from the knee crease on the inner side of the lower leg. This point regulates menstruation and the uterus, and is useful for irregular menstruation, impotence, and lower-back cramps during menstruation.

3. Hold SP6, the point that is three finger-widths up from the inner ankle, just behind the shinbone. This point is effective for bloating, fluid retention, abdominal cramps, and vaginal discharge. It can also help with insomnia, vertigo, and dizziness. Do not use this point if your partner is pregnant, as it can induce labor.

4. Hold LV3, the point in the webbing between the big toe and second toe. This point is helpful for cramping pain, breast tenderness, and emotional symptoms of PMS (including anger, frustration, hopelessness, and irritability).

Advanced Massage: Trigger Point Therapy (light to medium pressure, 2 to 3)

Warm up your partner's muscles using one or more of the basic massage techniques before moving on to trigger point therapy.

1. Uncover their leg and tuck the sheet under their other leg. Bend their leg at the knee and place it down with the sole of their foot on their other leg so that their inner thigh is exposed.

2. Find a spot on your partner's inner thigh (the **adductor** muscle) that causes pain (or that sends pain to another area of the body) when you press it. This sensation indicates a trigger point is present.

3. Use the trigger point therapy technique (page 27) on each spot on your partner's inner thigh that causes or refers pain.

Basic Massage: Kneading (light to medium pressure, 1 to 3)

For this technique, have your partner lie face down. Add lotion to your hands and rub them together to warm the lotion.

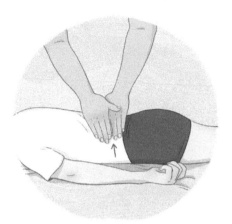

1. Move to one side of your partner. Press the heel of one hand into their lower back, and reach across with your other hand and pull their opposite side toward you, so you are lifting their lower back slightly between your hands. Rock their lower back between your hands as both hands glide toward their spine, releasing before they touch the spine.
2. Switch hands and repeat.
3. Reach across your partner's side with both hands and loosely hook your fingertips under their opposite side. Lean back, lifting their lower back and stretching the lower-back muscles you've hooked into. Using one hand at a time, hook your fingers under and slide your hand back toward you, replacing it with your other hand, which also slides back toward you. Repeat until the area loosens.
4. Switch sides and repeat Steps 2 to 4 on the other side of the lower back.

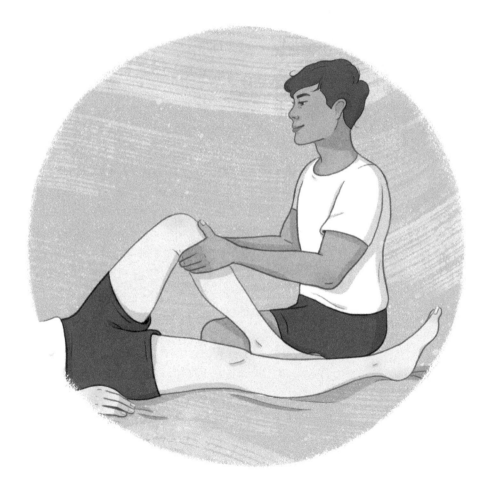

CHAPTER 8

Legs and Feet

Weekend warriors, office athletes, mall walkers, and everyone in between deals with sore feet and legs, as well as knee and ankle pain. This chapter provides a basic sequence plus basic and advanced massage techniques and tips to relieve pain from the following common ailments in our legs and feet.

LEGS AND FEET SEQUENCE

Basic Massage: Rocking and Shaking (light pressure, 1 to 2)

1. With your partner lying face down, start with one hand in a soft fist at their hip and the other hand pressing lightly at their lower leg. Lightly press down and move your hands away and then toward you at a pace that moves their whole leg. You can also use one hand on either side of their leg to rock it back and forth between your hands. Find your partner's rhythm and continue rocking for several minutes. As your partner relaxes, the rhythm may slow down.
2. Bend your partner's leg at the knee and hold their lower leg between your palms, moving your hands up and down the lower leg like you are starting a campfire.
3. Wrap your hands loosely around their ankle and shake their foot back and forth.
4. Turn your partner over so they are lying face up and rock their leg again, pinning at their hip and lower leg or rocking their leg between your hands.

For the following techniques, have your partner lie face down. Move the sheet to uncover your partner's leg and tuck it in between their legs. Add lotion to your hands and rub them together to warm the lotion.

Basic Massage: Gliding (light to medium pressure, 1 to 3)

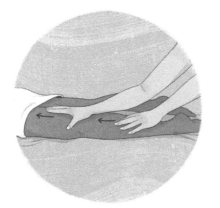

1. At your partner's side, place your hands palms down on their lower leg. Press your hands down, allowing your hands to follow the natural contours of their leg.
2. Glide your hands along your partner's leg with long, flowing strokes and slow, light pressure from their ankle up to their glutes. Repeat until their leg starts to feel soft and warm, adding more lotion as needed.

Basic Massage: Kneading (light to medium pressure, 1 to 3)

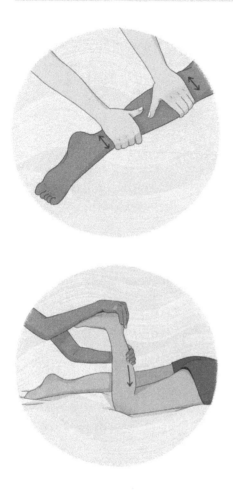

1. Still at their side, form a C with your hands and wrap the C around their lower leg (**calf muscles**), thumbs next to each other. Use both hands to slide the C along the lower leg, one hand at a time, in opposite directions (one hand up their leg, the other down their leg). Move your hands to the back of their upper leg (hamstrings) and repeat.

2. Press the heel of one hand into their lower calf and pull with the fingers of your other hand from the other side of their calf, alternating pushing and pulling as you move up to their knee and back down. Move your hands to the back of their upper leg and repeat.

3. Standing at your partner's feet, hold your partner's foot in both of your hands, using your thumbs to knead the sole of their foot.

4. From their side, bend your partner's leg at the knee and place the palm of one hand on their heel to hold the leg steady. Glide the other hand down their calf.

5. With their knee still bent, wrap your hands around their lower leg and glide your hands down their lower leg to their knee. Repeat, lowering their leg to the table as you finish and covering their leg with the sheet.

6. Repeat Steps 1 to 5 on the other leg.

Basic Massage: Rocking and Shaking (light pressure, 1 to 2)

With your partner lying face up, start with one hand in a soft fist at the hip and the other hand pressing lightly above the knee. Lightly press down and move your hands away and then toward you at a pace that moves their whole leg. You can also use one hand on either side of their leg to rock it back and forth between your hands. Find your partner's rhythm and continue rocking for several minutes. As your partner relaxes, the rhythm may slow down.

For the following techniques, have your partner lie face up. Move the sheet to uncover your partner's leg, then tuck it in between their legs. Add lotion to your hands and rub them together to warm the lotion.

Basic Massage: Gliding (light to medium pressure, 1 to 3)

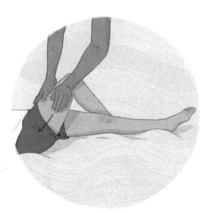

1. At your partner's side, place your hands palms down on their lower leg. Press your hands down, allowing your hands to follow the natural contours of their leg.
2. Glide your hands along your partner's leg with long, flowing strokes and slow, light pressure from the ankle up to the hip. Repeat until their leg starts to feel soft and warm, adding more lotion as needed.
3. Lift their knee and foot and plant the sole of their foot down on the table on the opposite side of their other knee. Move to the other side of the table and glide your hands from their knee to their hip.

Basic Massage: Kneading (light to medium pressure, 1 to 3)

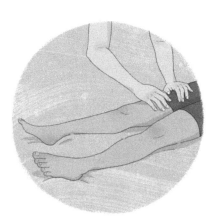

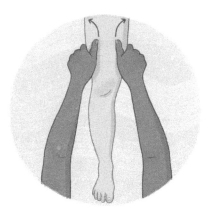

1. At your partner's side, form a C with your hands and wrap the C around the front of their lower leg, your thumbs next to each other. Use both hands to slide the C along the lower leg from ankle to knee, one hand at a time, in opposite directions (one hand up their leg, the other down their leg). Move your hands to their upper leg (the quadriceps muscle group, or "quads") and repeat.

2. At their knee, press the heel of one hand into their upper leg and pull with the fingers of your other hand from the other side of their upper leg, alternating pushing and pulling as you move up to their hip and back down.

3. With your hands on either side of their upper leg, use your thumb and index finger knuckle to knead the muscles from the center to the edges of the upper leg.

4. Bend their knee and bring the sole of their foot to the inside of their leg, exposing the inner thigh.

5. Face their feet and glide your hands from their knee to their hip.

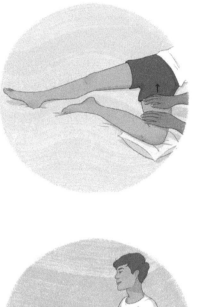

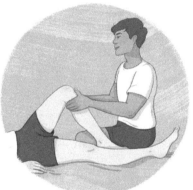

6. At their knee, press the heel of one hand into their inner thigh and pull with the fingers of your other hand from the back of their upper leg, alternating pushing and pulling as you move up to their hip and back down.

7. Lift their knee and place the sole of their foot flat on the table.

8. Sit on the table and wrap your hands around the lower leg, with your thumbs just below the knee.

9. Press your fingers into their calf muscles and pull your fingers toward the front of their leg, spreading their calf muscles apart.

10. Stand up and place their leg back on the table.

11. Hold their foot with both hands, with your thumbs on top of their foot.

12. Press your fingers into the center of the sole of their foot and pull your fingers out toward the sides, spreading their foot bones and pressing the top of their foot into your palms.

13. Rub each toe between your thumb and index finger knuckle from the base to the tip of their toe, pulling as you move toward the toenail.

14. Press the tip of each toe firmly between your thumb and index finger knuckle.

15. Repeat Steps 1 to 3 in the Gliding section as you finish.

SORE LEGS

Symptoms of sore legs include fatigue, weakness, wobbling, poor balance, heaviness in the legs, and swelling. Trigger points in the hamstrings, quadriceps, shins, and calves also cause achy soreness in the legs, along with pain in the groin or glutes, knee instability, calf cramping, and knee and foot pain. Massage can help by increasing circulation and lymph flow, flushing waste products out of tense and tired muscles at a faster rate than your body can on its own, speeding your recovery and increasing your strength and endurance. Massage also releases trigger points, relieving pain and restoring range of motion at your hips, knees, and ankles.

Basic Massage

1. Do the Hips sequence (page 114), paying special attention to the trigger points at the tops of the glutes along the hipbone.
2. Do the Legs and Feet sequence (page 132).

Basic Massage: Percussion (light pressure, 1 to 2)

Do not use percussion strokes right after exercising, as it may cause muscle cramps.

1. To energize your partner's leg muscles, turn them face up for percussion strokes.
2. With your hands facing each other, either open or in soft fists, lightly and quickly strike their upper leg muscles with the sides of your hands. Keep your fingers and wrists loose and move down their leg and back up (staying on the shin muscles and off the bone as you reach the lower leg).
3. With your hands cupped and facing downward, lightly and quickly strike their leg muscles with your hands, again moving from the upper leg down to the ankle and back up.
4. Turn your partner face down and repeat Steps 2 and 3 on the hamstrings and calf muscles, avoiding the backs of the knees.

Basic Massage: Acupressure (light pressure, 1 to 2)

1. Hold ST36, the point that is four finger-widths down from the outer side of the knee, just behind the shinbone (**tibia**). This point is helpful for poor circulation in the legs and leg muscle cramping and pain.
2. Hold ST40, the point that is midway between the knee and the ankle on the outer side of the leg, two finger-widths away from the side of the shinbone. This point is effective for cough, excessive phlegm, asthma, headache, dizziness, and weakness of the legs.
3. Hold the Huato 17 (see page 167) on the left side of the seventh thoracic vertebra, next to the spine at the same level as the pointy bottom of the shoulder blade. This point influences circulation and relieves swelling, weakness, and pain in the legs.

Advanced Massage: Friction (medium to firm pressure, 2 to 4)

Warm up your partner's muscles using one or more of the basic massage techniques before moving on to friction or trigger point therapy.

1. Find any taut bands of muscle tension that resist your pressure in your partner's leg.
2. Use the friction technique (page 26) to release any taut bands of muscle you find in the following areas:

   - The back of their upper leg (their hamstrings group).

   - Their calf muscles (**gastrocnemius** and **soleus**).

   - The front of their upper leg (their quadriceps muscles).

   - Your partner's shin muscle (**tibialis anterior**).

Advanced Massage: Trigger Point Therapy (medium to firm pressure, 2 to 4)

Warm up your partner's muscles using one or more of the basic massage techniques before moving on to trigger point therapy.

1. With your partner lying face down, find a spot on your partner's leg that causes pain (or that sends pain to another area of the body) when you press it. This sensation indicates a trigger point is present.

2. Use the trigger point therapy technique (page 27) on the following areas in your partner's legs that cause or refer pain:

    *   The muscles on the back of the leg above the inner and outer knee (the hamstrings).

    *   The muscles on the back of the leg below the inner and outer knee (the gastrocnemius).

    *   The small muscle on the back of the knee just below the knee crease (the **popliteus**).

    *   The deeper muscles on the lower half of the calf, particularly a few inches above the inner ankle (the soleus).

    *   The small thumb-sized muscle on the outer upper leg (the tensor fascia latae, which contracts to tighten the iliotibial band).

    *   The muscles on the inner thigh near the groin (the adductors).

    *   The big muscle on the front of the thigh that crosses from the upper leg to the hip-bone (the rectus femoris, one of the muscles in the quadriceps group).

    *   The thick muscle above the outside of the knee (the **vastus lateralis**, another muscle in the quadriceps group).

    *   The upper part of the muscle on the front of the shin (the tibialis anterior).

KNEE PAIN

Knee pain has many causes, partly due to its location between the ankle and hip, since issues in either joint also affect the knee. The four major muscle areas that affect the knee (the front and back of the upper and lower leg) each have their own potential issues that cause knee pain, along with possible injuries to the four ligaments that cross the knee and the cartilage inside. Knee pain can also be caused by arthritis, **gout**, or obesity.

Runner's knee is caused by tension in the **iliotibial band**, or **IT band**, the thick layer of fascia that stabilizes the upper leg and the quadriceps muscle group on the front of the upper leg. It connects to the front of the hip and runs down the side of the upper leg to the outer knee. When the quadriceps muscles are overworked, particularly the large muscle on the side of the upper leg (the **vastus lateralis**), the IT band can adhere to the muscles to provide extra stability. Unfortunately, these adhesions prevent the quadriceps muscles from working properly and cause pain and tension, especially on the outer edge of the knee.

There are four quadriceps muscles. They run from the upper leg to the knee, where they converge into a single tendon that runs across the knee to the shinbone. The kneecap (or **patella**) grows inside this tendon, so tension in the quadriceps muscles causes pain above, in, and below the knee.

On the back of the upper leg, the muscle group known as the **hamstrings** cross the knee to bend it. Tension in the hamstrings makes it difficult to straighten the leg, which draws the kneecap off its track and causes it to rub on the shinbone, which causes knee pain. The calf muscles also cross the back of the knee, so several trigger points in the surface calf muscle (the **gastrocnemius**) refer pain to the knee. A small muscle on the back of the knee (the **popliteus**) tightens when the knee is unstable, which also causes deep pain in the knee.

TIPS:

▶ If your partner has ligament or cartilage damage inside the knee, avoid moving their kneecap around, which might increase pain and inflammation inside their knee joint.

▶ For more lasting knee pain relief, incorporate regular stretches for your hamstrings, quadriceps, and calf muscles into your daily routine.

Basic Massage

1. Do the Legs and Feet sequence (page 132).
2. Do the friction and trigger point therapy techniques in the Sore Legs section (page 137), paying special attention to the taut bands and trigger points around the knee.

Basic Massage: Stretching

1. With your partner lying face up, stand at their side, facing their head. Bend their leg at the knee and hold their ankle with one hand.
2. Place your other hand on the back of their thigh under their knee.
3. Press their thigh and knee toward their chest to stretch the back of their upper leg (their hamstrings).
4. To increase the stretch, lift their lower leg and foot toward the ceiling, straightening their leg. Release gently and lower their leg to the table.
5. From your partner's side, face their feet. Hold your partner's heel with one hand and use your other hand to grip the top of their foot across the arch.
6. Press your partner's foot forward to point their toes and stretch the front of their foot and lower leg.
7. Bring your partner's foot back (toes to their nose) to stretch their heel and the calf muscles on their lower leg.
8. Tilt the edge of their foot inward, then outward, to stretch the sides of their lower leg.
9. With your partner lying face down, place your hand under their ankle. Bending their leg at the knee, bring their ankle to their glutes. To increase the stretch, put your knee on the table under their knee to lift their leg off the table. They should feel the stretch in the front of the hip and all along the quadriceps muscles, the quads.

Basic Massage: Acupressure (light pressure, 1 to 2)

1. Hold ST35, the point that is just below the kneecap on the outer side of the knee. This point relieves swelling and pain in the knee and restores knee mobility.
2. Hold GB34, the point on the side of the lower leg, about three finger-widths down from the knee and just behind the smaller lower leg bone (fibula). This point is useful for numbness and pain in the legs, swelling and pain in the knee, shoulder pain, and joint and ligament issues.
3. Hold UB40, the point on the back of the knee between the tendons on the outer edge of the knee. This point increases blood flow to the knee and relieves sciatic pain.

ANKLE PAIN

85 percent of ankle pain is caused by a sprain (an overstretched or torn ligament in the ankle), which can cause pain, bruising, swelling, and ankle instability. Ankle pain may also result from arthritis in the foot, wear and tear on the ankle joints, improper shoes, **sciatica**, obesity, or **gout** (a buildup of uric acid in the body that deposits crystals in the joints, which cause pain and swelling).

Massage can help by preventing scar tissue from forming after an ankle sprain. It can also relieve tight muscles in the lower leg and foot, reduce swelling, aid in waste removal, and speed recovery.

> TIP:
> ▶ Wait at least 72 hours before massaging your partner's ankle after a sprain. Avoid any inflamed areas (swollen, soft, and squishy, and possibly red or warm to the touch).

Basic Massage

Do the Legs and Feet sequence (page 132), paying extra attention to your partner's lower leg and foot.

Basic Massage: Stretching

1. From your partner's side, face their feet. Hold your partner's heel with one hand and use the other hand to grip the top of their foot across the arch.
2. Press your partner's foot forward to point their toes and stretch the front of their foot.
3. Bring your partner's foot back (toes to their nose) to stretch the heel and bottom of their foot.
4. Tilt the edge of their foot inward, then outward, to stretch the sides of their foot.

Basic Massage: Acupressure (light pressure, 1 to 2)

1. Hold KI6, the point that is one finger-width below the inner ankle. This point is effective for swollen and stiff ankles.
2. Hold GB40, the point that is just in front of the outer ankle. This point relieves pain from sprains, swelling, and sciatic pain in the foot.
3. Hold UB60, the point that is just behind the outer ankle, next to the heel tendon. This point is helpful for swollen feet, pain in the lower back, thigh, and ankle, and arthritis in the foot.

Advanced Massage: Friction (medium to firm pressure, 2 to 4)

Warm up your partner's muscles using one or more of the basic massage techniques before moving on to friction.

1. Find the taut ligament band that your partner sprained in their ankle.
2. Using stacked hands or fingers or supported thumbs, press the pads of your fingers into their ligament perpendicularly (so your pressure is directed into and across their ligament).
3. Firmly and quickly press your fingers across their ankle ligament, alternating strokes along the ligament in one direction (across the ligament).
4. Next, find a taut band of muscle tension that resists your pressure in the side of their lower leg (their **peroneus** group of muscles).
5. Use the friction technique (page 26) to release any taut bands of muscle in their lower leg.

Advanced Massage: Trigger Point Therapy (medium to firm pressure, 2 to 4)

Warm up your partner's muscles using one or more of the basic massage techniques before moving on to trigger point therapy.

1. With your partner lying face up, find a spot on their lower leg that causes pain (or that sends pain to another area of the body) when you press it. This sensation indicates a trigger point is present.
2. Use the trigger point therapy technique (page 27) on the following areas in your partner's lower leg that cause or refer pain:

    - The muscles on the side of their lower leg, about four finger-widths down from their knee and four finger-widths up from their ankle (the peroneus group of muscles).

SORE FEET

Achy feet make it difficult to get to all the places you need to go every day. This can be caused by standing too long, walking long distances (particularly on uneven ground), wearing shoes without proper fit or support, and dealing with injuries to your foot and ankle.

Massage can help by relaxing the tense muscles in your feet, increasing circulation, reducing swelling, and relieving pain. Massage also releases trigger points in foot muscles, eliminating the source of dull, achy pain referral patterns and restoring full range of motion to your foot and ankle. Your foot has more than 200,000 nerve endings, so reflexology and acupressure in the foot can relieve aches and pains all over the body (which may be causing your foot soreness in a particular spot).

TIPS:

▶ To relieve achy feet quickly, soak your feet in a basin of warm water and Epsom salts, which relaxes the muscles and fascia in your foot and restores magnesium to your cells (an important nutrient for proper muscle function).

▶ Roll a tennis ball under your foot to relieve stiff and aching feet and allow your foot to relax and spread out on the floor. Start and end by rolling the ball from toes to heel. Hold the ball under your toes, under the ball of your foot, and under your heel, putting your weight into the ball as if you want to pop it. Don't forget the inner and outer edges of your foot!

▶ **Essential oils:** Peppermint and eucalyptus essential oils are invigorating for sore muscles. Try adding a few drops to your lotion or oil to energize your partner's sore feet. (See page 48 for notes on essential oil safety.)

Basic Massage

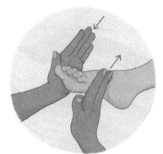

1. With your partner lying face up, kneel at their feet. (You can use lotion here if you want to, but it isn't necessary if your partner doesn't like it.)
2. Hold their foot with both your hands and move your hands up and down the sides of their foot like you are starting a campfire, rocking the foot between your hands.
3. Hold their foot at the inside of their arch with one hand.
4. Wrap your other hand around the base of the toes and rotate the foot outward, pressing in with your other thumb at the arch of their foot.
5. While continuing to hold their arch with your thumb, use your hand on top of their foot to cover their toes and pull them toward their nose, pressing into the top of their arch with your other thumb.

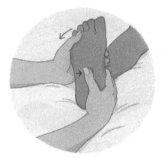

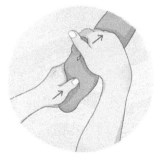

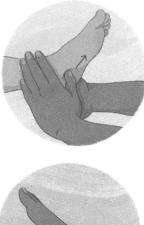

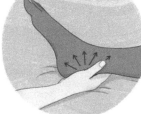

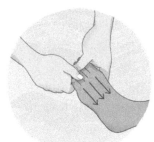

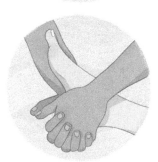

6. With both of your thumbs on the sole of their foot, knead their sole from heel to toe, allowing your thumbs to follow the natural arches of their foot.

7. Hold their heel in the palm of your hand and stroke the thick tendon at the back of their heel (the **calcaneal tendon**) with your thumb in all directions, making a sunray pattern.

8. Stand at your partner's feet and face the head of the table. Hold their foot in both of your hands with your thumbs on top of their foot.

9. Glide your thumbs into the webbing between each of the tendons for the toes, from the base of the toes up to the front of the ankle.

10. Holding their foot with one hand, pinch the sides of each toe firmly with your other thumb and index finger, above and below their toe knuckle, holding for a few seconds in each spot.

11. Pinch the tips of each toe firmly, holding for a few seconds.

12. Turn so you are facing their feet from the side of the table and clasp your partner's heel between your hands, interlacing your fingers at the back of the heel.

13. Press your palms together firmly. Release gently.

Basic Massage: Percussion (light pressure, 1 to 2)

Holding your partner's toes back with one hand, lightly and quickly strike the sole of the foot with the side of your other hand, keeping your fingers and wrist loose.

Basic Massage: Acupressure (light pressure, 1 to 3)

1. Hold UB60, the point just behind the outer ankle, next to the heel tendon. This point is helpful for swollen feet, pain in the lower back, thigh, and ankle, and arthritis in the foot.
2. Hold UB62, the point just below the outer anklebone. This point is useful for heel pain, ankle pain, aching feet, and insomnia.

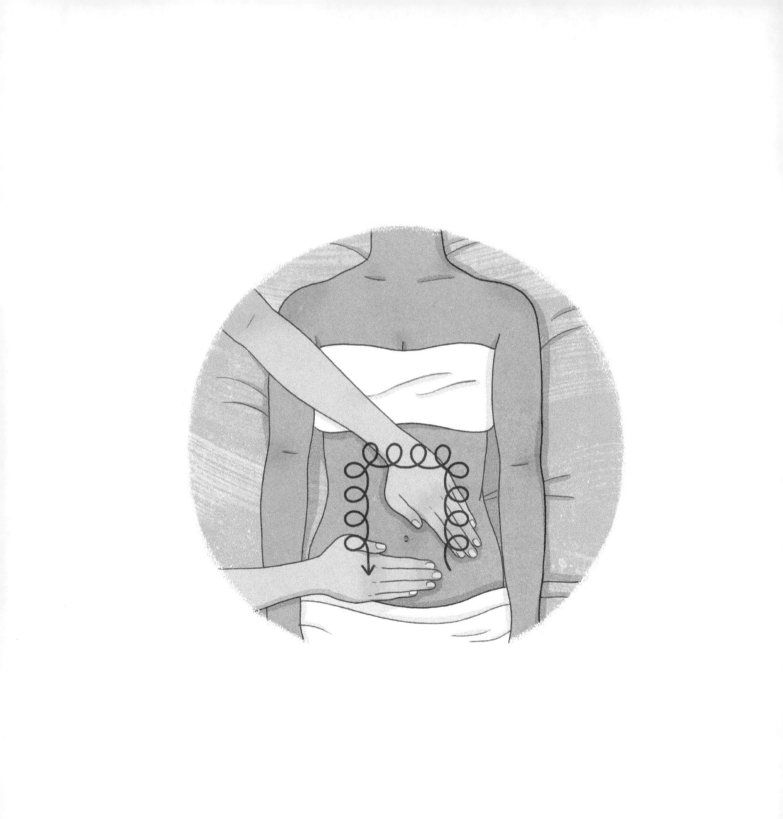

CHAPTER 9

Full-Body Ailments

In our culture of chronic stress, we often deal with chronic pain and illness. Massage therapy is not only useful for physical relief, but it has also been used to address mental health in cultures around the world for centuries. Health-care professionals are recommending massage therapy to treat mental health issues more than ever before. This chapter provides basic and advanced massage techniques and tips to relieve symptoms of the following full-body ailments and mental health issues.

PAINFUL JOINTS AND ARTHRITIS

Nearly 46 million adults suffer from some form of arthritis that limits their daily functions. In common **osteoarthritis**, cartilage on the ends of bones inside the joint wears away due to overuse, leaving the bones exposed to friction and causing rough bony surfaces to develop. This type of arthritis is typically joint-specific. Massage cannot help heal this condition; unfortunately, cartilage doesn't grow back. However, massage *can* loosen tight muscles around the joint that are pulling the rough bony surfaces together, which will decrease pain and inflammation within the joint.

Less commonly, **rheumatoid arthritis** involves inflammation of the fibrous connective tissue around joints and is typically body-wide. This condition is not well understood; studies suggest it may be an **autoimmune disorder** (when the body attacks its own cells because it cannot recognize them properly), a hormonal or glandular imbalance, or it could even be related to viral infections. If your partner is diagnosed with rheumatoid arthritis, consult with their doctor before doing massage, and never give them a massage during a flare-up (when they can scarcely bear to be touched).

TIPS:

▶ Basic Swedish and acupressure massage have been proven to be most beneficial for painful joints, as deeper techniques can increase inflammation in sensitive, swollen joints. Avoid inflamed areas (swollen, soft, and squishy, and possibly red or warm to the touch) and use a light touch. Just providing a relaxing massage that increases circulation will be wonderful relief for your partner.

▶ As my chiropractor says, motion is lotion for the joints! The more you move, the more fluid is produced inside the joints to cushion and repair them. Increase your physical activity, daily and across the week, to your pain tolerance. Make sure to rest well between sessions.

▶ Reduce your weight with a healthy anti-inflammatory diet, frequent exercise, high water intake (at least half an ounce for every pound you weigh), and proper sleep (6 to 8 hours or more). Every four pounds you lose decreases the load on your knee and ankle joints.

▶ **Essential oils:** To further relieve joint pain, add your own blend of healing essential oils to your massage lotion. Try wintergreen or birch (see safety note, page 49), peppermint, eucalyptus, thyme, or cinnamon.

Another less common condition is **gout**, which also causes pain in the joints. This is a buildup of uric acid in the body that deposits crystals in the joints, which causes swelling and chronic joint pain. Avoid your partner's joints if they have been diagnosed with gout, as massage will grind the crystals together. As with osteoarthritis, however, massage can help loosen tight muscles around gouty joints, reducing pain and inflammation.

For all three conditions, massage can help by easing muscle tension and stiffness, improving circulation, reducing swelling, and improving joint mobility and grip strength. It also increases immune function and the body's production of endorphins (the hormones that enable you to endure pain better). Massage also relieves symptoms of arthritis, like insomnia, anxiety, stress, fatigue, and depression.

Basic Massage

1. Do the Head, Neck, and Chest sequence (page 60).
2. Do the Back and Shoulders sequence (page 84).
3. Do the Arms and Hands sequence (page 102).
4. Do the Hips sequence (page 114).
5. Do the Legs and Feet sequence (page 132).

Basic Massage: Acupressure (light pressure, 1 to 2)

1. Hold LI11, the point on back of the forearm at the edge of the elbow crease. This point relieves arthritic pain, especially in the elbow and shoulder, and diarrhea, constipation, and abdominal pain.
2. Hold TH5, the point that is three finger-widths down from the wrist on the back of the forearm. This point is useful for rheumatism, tendonitis, wrist pain, and shoulder pain.
3. Hold GB24, the point on the outside of the lower leg that is just behind the top (head) of the smaller lower leg bone (fibula). This point is effective for pain of the shoulder, arthritis, weakness, numbness and pain of the lower extremities, and swelling and pain of the knee.

POOR CIRCULATION

Poor circulation has many causes, including **atherosclerosis** (plaque buildup in the arteries), diabetes-related nerve damage, blood clots, obesity, and tobacco smoking. People with poor circulation have a wide variety of symptoms, including numbness, tingling, and cold in the hands and feet, swelling in the feet, ankles, and legs (due to fluid pooling in the area, called **edema**), fatigue, muscle cramping, memory loss, difficulty concentrating, digestive issues, leg or foot ulcers, and varicose veins.

Massage can help by improving circulation and metabolism, decreasing stress, enhancing sleep, and encouraging fluid drainage to reduce swelling.

TIPS:

▶ Basic Swedish and acupressure massage have been proven to be most beneficial for poor circulation, as deeper techniques can be painful in cold areas and can increase swelling. Avoid inflamed areas (swollen, soft, and squishy, and possibly red or warm to the touch) and use a light touch. Just providing a relaxing massage that increases circulation will be wonderful relief for your partner.

▶ Movement pumps blood and lymph circulation, particularly in the legs and feet, which rely on the walking movements of the deep lower-leg muscle (the **soleus**) to return blood to the heart; that's why they also call the soleus the "second heart"! Increase your physical activity, daily and across the week, to your pain tolerance. Make sure to rest well between sessions.

▶ Try a cayenne balm or capsicum lotion on areas with poor circulation. You can also try turmeric or glucosamine chondroitin supplements, which are often used for their anti-inflammatory benefits.

▶ There are "massage shoes" you can obtain, which have small stones or plastic pegs inside the shoe where the sole of your foot rests. If your doctor okays it, grab a pair to stimulate circulation in your feet as you walk during the day.

▶ Use the Legs Up the Wall yoga pose to allow gravity to return fluid to the torso. Lie on the floor and lift your legs up perpendicular to the floor, at a 90-degree angle to the body. You can also sit sideways with your hip at a wall, then turn the front of your body toward the wall, swinging your legs up the wall as you lie back on the floor. Either way, hold for a few minutes, then bend your knees and bring your legs down, releasing slowly to the floor or turning to your side.

▶ **Essential oils:** Warming oils like ginger or clove can boost circulation when added to your massage lotion or oil. (See page 48 for notes on essential oil safety.)

Basic Massage

1. Do the Head, Neck, and Chest sequence (page 60).
2. Do the Back and Shoulders sequence (page 84).
3. Do the Arms and Hands sequence (page 102).
4. Do the Hips sequence (page 114).
5. Do the Legs and Feet sequence (page 132).

Basic Massage: Acupressure (light pressure, 1 to 2)

1. Hold SP10, the point that is two finger-widths up from the kneecap on the center of the inner thigh (when the knee is bent). This point is known as the Sea of Blood and is the go-to point for blood disorders, as it regulates blood circulation and menstruation, particularly circulation in the legs.
2. Hold ST36, the point that is four finger-widths down from the outer side of the knee, just behind the shinbone (tibia). This point is helpful for poor circulation in the legs, leg-muscle cramping and pain, depression, anxiety, fatigue, digestive issues, chronic illness, and decreased immune function.
3. Hold LV3, the point in the webbing between the big toe and the second toe. This point is helpful for regulating blood circulation and menstruation, relieving headaches, vertigo, and hiccups, decreasing leg muscle cramping and pain, weakness, and numbness, and improving emotional symptoms, like anger, frustration, depression, and irritability.

MUSCLE CRAMPS

Muscle cramps are an unpleasant, painful sensation caused by an involuntary muscle contraction. When a muscle cramps, it suddenly hardens by itself and will not release. You can see and feel the tight contraction in your partner's muscle. Muscle cramps can be caused by dehydration, muscle fatigue or overuse, heart or liver disease, diabetes, nerve damage, pregnancy, obesity, low **electrolytes**, or prescription medications.

TIPS:

▶ Do not use percussion, friction, or trigger point therapy on your partner after an athletic event or a hard workout, as these quick or deep techniques can cause muscle cramps.

▶ Increase your water intake to at least half an ounce for every pound you weigh (so if you weigh 200 pounds, you should drink at least 100 ounces of water daily).

▶ Ensure that you take in enough **electrolytes** (which include sodium, potassium, and magnesium, elements that are essential to muscle function), either through food and water or by adding a vitamin supplement. You can also take warm Epsom salt baths to absorb magnesium through your skin and relieve tension in areas that cramp regularly.

Basic Massage: During a Muscle Cramp

1. Move quickly—your partner is in a lot of pain!
2. Place your stacked hands over the area that is cramping and hold firm pressure (3 to 4) for at least a minute or until the cramp releases. If that doesn't work, go to Step 3.
3. Have them stretch the muscle that is cramping by shortening the opposite muscle. Make sure they do the move, not you, because the opposite muscle will only contract when they move it.
4. Here is a list to help a cramping muscle—tell your partner to do the following for the applicable body area:

   • Neck, both sides: "Bring your chin to your chest."

   • Neck, one side: "Bring your ear or nose to your shoulder on the opposite side."

   • Chest: "Move your shoulder blades together."

   • Upper and middle back: "Bring your elbows together in front of your chest."

   • Lower back, both sides: "Do a forward bend at your waist." Or: "Do a slight crunch with your abs."

   • Lower back, one side: "Bend sideways to your opposite side, sliding your hand down your pants seam."

   • Biceps: "Straighten your arm."

- Triceps: "Bring your fist to your shoulder."

- Glutes: "Bring your knee to your opposite shoulder."

- Quads: "Bring your heel to your glutes."

- Hamstrings: "Bring your knee to your chest, pointing your toes toward your nose."

- Calf: "Point your toes toward your nose."

- Shin: "Point your toes and turn them inward."

- Sole of foot: "Point your toes toward your nose."

5. Once the cramp has stopped, you can stretch the muscle that was cramping, using the basic massage stretching techniques in the area where your partner's muscle cramped. For stretching, you perform the move, not your partner.
6. Use cold compresses or ice to soothe your partner's pain after a muscle cramp.

Basic Massage: After a Muscle Cramp

1. Use a hot towel or hot stones on the area where your partner's muscle cramped.
2. Do any basic massage, stretching, or acupressure techniques in the area where your partner's muscle cramped, or hold the following acupressure points.

Basic Massage: Acupressure (light pressure, 1 to 2)

1. Hold GV26, the point that is directly in the crease below the nose. This point relieves muscle cramps, dizziness, and fainting.
2. Hold UB57, the point on the back of the leg in the center of the calf muscle (**gastrocnemius**) that is halfway between the crease of the knee and the heel. This point is useful for muscle cramps, especially those occurring in the legs, as well as knee pain, lower-back pain, and swelling in the feet.
3. Hold ST36, the point that is four finger-widths down from the outer side of the knee, just behind the shinbone (tibia). This point is helpful for leg-muscle cramping.

DIGESTIVE ISSUES

Many circumstances contribute to digestive issues, particularly in our culture of chronic stress. When we are in our fight-flight-or-freeze response, digestive functions are slowed to increase blood flow to the limbs and respiratory system. If we live in chronic stress, we struggle constantly with digesting and eliminating, which manifests as **irritable bowel syndrome** (IBS), heartburn, nausea, gas, intestinal inflammation, diarrhea, constipation, and food sensitivities. Poor diet and nutrition, dehydration, and lack of exercise also cause chronic digestive issues.

There are also chronic autoimmune disorders that affect the digestive tract, including **ulcerative colitis** (inflammation of the lining of the colon) and **Crohn's disease** (inflammation of the lining of the entire digestive tract). These disorders (sometimes are referred to together as **inflammatory bowel disease**, or IBD) typically include symptoms like bloody diarrhea, rectal bleeding and pain, colon inflammation, abdominal pain, intestinal cramping, low iron, chronic fatigue, and weight loss.

Massage can help by relaxing the body and stimulating elimination, reducing constipation, and decreasing the time between bowel movements. Massage may also reduce bloating, aid in weight loss, increase blood flow to the abdomen, and tone and strengthen the abdominal muscles. Trigger points in the lower back and belly can cause digestive issues, so releasing those points can relieve symptoms.

> TIPS:
>
> ▶ Practice mindful eating. Turn off electronics, sit at a table, and chew your food carefully. Taste and enjoy what you are eating. Take sips of water between bites. Eat slowly and listen for your body's cues that you are full.
>
> ▶ If your digestive issues continue, keep a journal of your symptoms, food and water intake, activities, and stress levels to determine the triggers for your condition.
>
> ▶ **Essential oils:** To further ease digestive upset, add your own blend of soothing essential oils to your massage lotion or use a diffuser to scent the room. Try ginger, peppermint, black pepper, or lemongrass. (See page 48 for notes on essential oil safety.)

Basic Massage

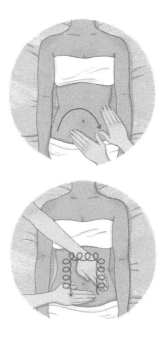

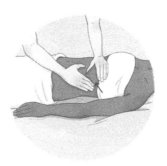

1. Have your partner lie face up. From their right side, touch their arm and shoulder first to introduce your touch.
2. Gently place your hands on their stomach with your palms down. You can add lotion to your hands now if they are unclothed, rubbing your hands together to warm the lotion.
3. Press your hands gently into the stomach and circle them over the belly button, finding a soft rhythm.
4. Starting at your partner's lower left side (near where the colon empties into the rectum), make small friction circles with your fingertips, up to their ribs, across to their right side, and down to their right side. This movement encourages elimination in the colon.
5. Place one hand over your partner's ribs on one side, and press your fingertips on your other hand underneath the ribs.

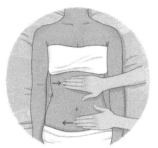

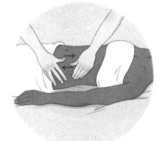

6. Make small friction circles underneath your partner's ribs from the center of their belly out to the side of their body.

7. Place one hand just under your partner's ribs and your other hand below the belly button. Slowly pull your top hand toward you and press your lower hand away from you, pressing into the belly to stimulate movement in your partner's colon.

8. With C-shaped hands, gently grasp and lift the left side of your partner's belly.

9. Repeat on their right side.

10. Finish with soft belly circles as in Step 3.

Basic Massage: Acupressure

1. Hold LI4, the point on the back of the hand in the webbing where the thumb and index finger meet. Avoid this point if your partner is pregnant, as it can induce labor. This point relieves pain of all kinds and improves waste elimination and constipation.

2. Hold two points at the same time: PC6, the point that is three finger-widths down from the crease of the wrist on the inner forearm, in the center between the two thickest tendons, along with TH5, the point that is three finger-widths down from the wrist on the back of the forearm. When held together, these points influence the immune system, build resistance to infection, and relieve stomachache, indigestion, nausea, vomiting, and anxiety.

3. Hold CV6, the point that is two finger-widths down from the belly button on the center of the abdomen. This point is helpful for gas, irritable bowel syndrome, headache, and general weakness. It can also relieve irregular periods, menstrual cramps, and vaginal discharge.

4. Hold LI11, the point on back of the forearm at the edge of the elbow crease. This point relieves arthritic pain, especially in the elbow and shoulder, and diarrhea, constipation, and abdominal pain.

5. Hold SP4, the point on the arch of the foot that is just below the ball of the foot, in line with the big toe. This point relieves gastric pain and bloating, poor appetite, indigestion, nausea, and diarrhea.

STRESS AND ANXIETY

Stress is any situation that requires a response from the body or brain. It is a natural part of life. Healthy reactions to stress help us interact with our environment and maintain our physical and emotional balance. What we call stress is actually *distress*—a set of negative reactions to chronic stress, which can include depression, anxiety, headaches, nausea, high blood pressure, difficulty sleeping, or sexual dysfunction.

Distress can also appear as chronic pain, fatigue, gastrointestinal issues, weakened immune system, changes in weight and appetite, muscle tension, and a host of other issues that make a person's underlying condition difficult to diagnose and treat. In fact, stress is linked to six of the leading causes of death in the United States: heart disease, cancer, lung ailments, accidents, cirrhosis of the liver, and suicide.

Anxiety is the body's natural response to stress—a nagging feeling of fear or worry about the future. These feelings naturally come and go as our circumstances change. If they persist for more than six months and interfere with your ability to function daily, you may be dealing with an anxiety disorder, such as **generalized anxiety disorder**, which affects over 6.8 millions American adults. Symptoms of GAD include nervousness, irritability, increased heart rate, rapid breathing, fatigue, insomnia, difficulty concentrating, muscle tension, and digestive issues. GAD often affects people dealing with chronic pain and other chronic health issues.

Thankfully, just one 60-minute massage session has been shown to decrease stress hormone levels by 30 percent (cortisol) and increase pain-relieving hormone levels by 28 percent (serotonin) and 31 percent (dopamine). These changes allow your body to shift out of its chronic stress response, boosting relaxation and pain relief and allowing you to release anxious or fearful thoughts and respond to triggers in an intentional, healthy way.

- ▶ To ease the high energy of stress and anxiety, start with faster movements, like rocking and shaking and work down to slower, more meditative movements, like feathering and acupressure.

- ▶ Encourage your partner to avoid talking about or thinking about stressful matters, including work, family, health, or money issues, during your massage session. Use this time to practice healthy coping skills: for example, meditation, prayer, or visualization.

- ▶ **Essential oils:** For additional anxiety relief, add your own blend of anxiety-relieving essential oils to your massage lotion or use a diffuser to scent the room. Try bergamot, lavender, geranium, sandalwood, cedarwood, cypress, ylang ylang, vetiver, frankincense, or marjoram. (See page 48 for notes on essential oil safety.)

Basic Massage

1. Do rocking and shaking for the whole body (back, arms, and legs).
2. Do the Head, Neck, and Chest sequence (page 60).
3. Do the Back and Shoulders sequence (page 84).
4. Do the Arms and Hands sequence (page 102).
5. Do the Hips sequence (page 114).
6. Do the Legs and Feet sequence (page 132).
7. If your partner's anxiety is the result of chronic pain, try the other basic and advanced techniques for that area as well.

Basic Massage: Feathering (light pressure, 1)

Using both hands, stroke from the base of the head to the base of the spine with rhythmic movements (see page 29). As one hand reaches the bottom of the spine, the other hand starts at the neck, so there is always one hand moving down the spine. Use this stroke for at least three minutes to reset and sedate the nervous system.

Basic Massage: Acupressure (light pressure, 1 to 2)

1. Hold GB20, the point that is just below the base of the head on either side of the neck, about two finger-widths away from the spine. This point reduces stress, calms the mind, improves breathing, and helps with headaches and neck and jaw pain. It also helps with insomnia, fatigue, and general irritability.

2. Hold UB15, the point that is one finger-width from the spine at the midpoint between the top and bottom points of the shoulder blade. This point is effective for relieving chest pain, heart palpitations, chest congestion, difficulty breathing, forgetfulness, and symptoms of anxiety and insomnia.

3. Hold PC6, the point that is three finger-widths down from the crease of the wrist on the inner forearm, in the center between the two thickest tendons. This point relieves pain and fullness in the chest, anxiety, depression, insomnia, nausea, motion sickness, and wrist pain.

4. Hold HT7, the point that is on the pinky side of the inner wrist crease, just inside the nearest tendon to the edge. This point is helpful for chest pain, irregular heart rate, insomnia, and forgetfulness. It is known as the main point for emotional issues, especially anxiety and worry.

INSOMNIA AND FATIGUE

Insomnia means difficulty sleeping, whether falling asleep, staying asleep, or waking up in the morning. It has many causes, including emotional and mental health issues, excessive eating or exercising, alcohol or drug use, chronic illness, and pain. Symptoms of insomnia also include headache, dizziness, irregular heart rate, fatigue, forgetfulness, and anxiety. Chronic insomnia affects your concentration, mood, reaction time, and work performance. It also puts you at higher risk for obesity, heart disease, and substance abuse.

Fatigue is typically used to describe the feeling of being extremely tired, both physically and mentally, for a prolonged period of time. Mental fatigue includes difficulty concentrating and learning new tasks, daytime sleepiness, irritability, and poor decision-making skills. Physical fatigue includes exhaustion, muscle weakness, headaches, digestive issues, vision problems, and inability to do physical tasks, like climbing stairs.

When fatigue is caused by poor sleep, it can be associated with diabetes, high blood pressure, heart disease, obesity, and depression. Fatigue can also be caused by a lack of iron in the blood (**anemia**), thyroid conditions, diabetes, lung and heart conditions, mental health issues, hormonal imbalances, drug side effects, allergens, vitamin deficiencies, and obesity.

Chronic Fatigue Syndrome, or CFS, is tiredness that is unrelated to the amount of sleep you get. Symptoms can include memory loss, insomnia, reduced mobility, headaches, anxiety, depression, and chronic pain. When this condition is severe, it affects your ability to go to school or work.

Massage can help with insomnia and fatigue by stimulating hormones, like endorphins and serotonin, to improve your mood and increase your energy level. Massage increases circulation, which alleviates numbness, weakness, and sluggishness. Massage also relieves stress, anxiety, and pain, which contribute to insomnia and fatigue. Finally, bedtime massage improves the quality and length of your sleep by increasing serotonin levels, an essential hormone for melatonin production (which regulates your awake and sleep cycles).

TIPS:

▶ To relieve the low energy of insomnia and fatigue, start your massage with slower movements, like acupressure and gliding, and work your way up to faster, more energizing movements (if your partner can handle them).

▶ Slow, gentle massage may be necessary if your partner's fatigue causes sensitivity to pressure and speed, so start with light pressure.

▶ Schedule your massage session right before bedtime so your partner can transition smoothly into sleep from your massage. If possible, do your session with your partner on the bed so they can fall asleep as you massage. Incorporating a short massage session into your partner's daily bedtime routine can help signal their body that it is time for sleep.

▶ **Essential oils:**

• To improve sleep, add your own blend of restful essential oils to your massage lotion or use a diffuser to scent the room. Try geranium, chamomile, cedarwood, vetiver, clary sage, or lavender. Do not use clary sage if you or your partner are pregnant!

• To stimulate wakefulness, add your own blend of invigorating essential oils to your massage lotion or use a diffuser. Try cypress, rosemary, lemongrass, ginger, black pepper, or any citrus oil. (See page 48 for notes on essential oil safety.)

Basic Massage

1. Do the Head, Neck, and Chest sequence (page 60).
2. Do the Back and Shoulders sequence (page 84).
3. Do the Arms and Hands sequence (page 102).
4. Do the Hips sequence (page 114).
5. Do the Legs and Feet sequence (page 132).
6. If your partner's insomnia is caused by chronic pain or stiffness, try the other basic and advanced techniques for that area as well.

Basic Massage: Feathering (light pressure, 1)

Have your partner lie face down. Using both hands, stroke from the base of your partner's head to the base of their spine with rhythmic movements. As one hand reaches the bottom of the spine, your other hand starts at their neck, so there is always one hand moving down their spine. Use this stroke for at least 3 minutes to reset and sedate your partner's nervous system.

Basic Massage: Acupressure (light pressure, 1 to 3)

1. Hold UB15, the point that is one finger-width from the spine at the midpoint between the top and bottom points of the shoulder blade. This point is effective for relieving chest pain, heart palpitations, chest congestion, difficulty breathing, forgetfulness, and symptoms of anxiety and insomnia.
2. Hold ST36, the point that is four finger-widths down from the outer side of the knee, just behind the shinbone (tibia). This point is helpful for poor circulation in the legs, leg muscle cramping and pain, depression, anxiety, fatigue, digestive issues, chronic illness, and decreased immune function.
3. Hold HT7, the point that is on the pinky side of the inner wrist crease, just inside the nearest tendon to the edge. This point is helpful for chest pain, irregular heart rate, forgetfulness, and symptoms of insomnia and anxiety. It is known as the main point for emotional issues, especially excessive worry and anxiety.
4. Hold KI1, the point that is at the center of the ball of the foot, where the sole of the foot creases when the toes are curled. This point is calming and induces restful sleep.

DEPRESSION

Depression is characterized by emotional and social withdrawal, prolonged sadness and hopelessness, loss of interest in your favorite things, and sometimes even thoughts of harming yourself. Other symptoms include irritability, restlessness, fatigue, low energy, difficulty concentrating, insomnia, changes in your appetite, chronic pain, cramps, or digestive problems, and feeling guilty, worthless, or helpless. Chronic depression is usually diagnosed when you have dealt with five or more of these symptoms over a two-week period or longer.

Depression can be caused by sudden changes in your physical or emotional circumstances, including changes in your relationships, finances, or career. If you deal with depression, you are not alone. Depression affects 10 percent of American adults and can cause chronic pain, asthma, heart disease, diabetes, and obesity. It also costs you money when you miss work, go on short-term disability, or feel unproductive.

Massage can help by improving your mood through increased serotonin levels. Studies have shown that regular massage sessions over several weeks can significantly reduce the severity and number of your symptoms of depression.

TIPS:

▶ To relieve the low energy of depression, start with slower movements, like acupressure and gliding, and work your way up to faster, more energizing movements, like percussion.

▶ Reach out. Find a friend, family member, colleague, or health professional to talk to about your feelings of isolation, sadness, and hopefulness. Learn positive coping skills and break unhealthy thought patterns and habits. You are worth the time and effort to get help. Only you can serve your unique purpose in this world!

▶ Get active. Add a little bit of movement each day, whether it's taking the stairs, checking the mail, taking a walk, or going to the gym. It all adds up, and a tiny bit is better than nothing. Better yet if you get some sun, which increases serotonin levels and boosts your mood.

▶ **Essential oils:** To increase the antidepressant effect, add your own blend of uplifting essential oils to your massage lotion or use a diffuser to scent the room. Try eucalyptus, cypress, frankincense, lemongrass, lime, peppermint, black pepper, rosemary, thyme, ginger, or any citrus oil.

Basic Massage

1. Do the Head, Neck, and Chest sequence (page 60).
2. Do the Back and Shoulders sequence (page 84).
3. Do the Arms and Hands sequence (page 102).
4. Do the Hips sequence (page 114).
5. Do the Legs and Feet sequence (page 132).
6. If your partner's depression is the result of chronic pain, arthritis, or fatigue, also try the other basic and advanced techniques for that area or ailment.

Basic Massage: Percussion (light pressure, 1 to 2)

Do percussion over the entire body with your partner lying faceup and face down.

Basic Massage: Acupressure (light pressure, 1 to 2)

1. Hold CV17, the point that is in the center of the chest, on the breastbone between the pectoral muscles. This point relieves chest pain, difficulty breathing, and symptoms of depression.
2. Hold ST36, the point that is four finger-widths down from the outer side of the knee, just behind the shinbone (tibia). This point is helpful for poor circulation in the legs, leg muscle cramping and pain, depression, anxiety, fatigue, digestive issues, chronic illness, and decreased immune function.
3. Hold LV3, the point in the webbing between the big toe and the second toe. This point is helpful for regulating blood circulation and menstruation, relieving headaches, vertigo, and hiccups, decreasing leg muscle cramping and pain, weakness, and numbness, and improving emotional symptoms like anger, frustration, depression, and irritability.

Acupressure Points

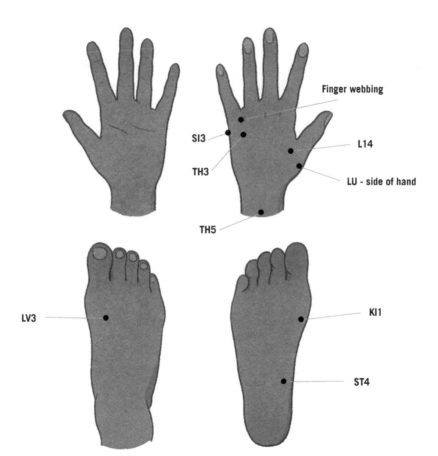

Finger webbing

SI3

TH3

L14

LU - side of hand

TH5

LV3

KI1

ST4

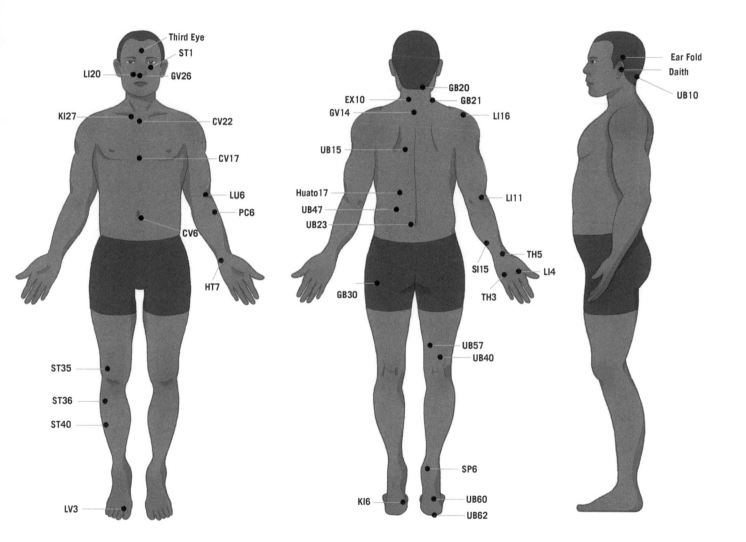

Third Eye
ST1
LI20
GV26
KI27
CV22
CV17
LU6
PC6
CV6
HT7
ST35
ST36
ST40
LV3

EX10
GB20
GV14
GB21
LI16
UB15
Huato17
UB47
UB23
LI11
SI15
TH5
LI4
TH3
GB30
UB57
UB40
SP6
KI6
UB60
UB62

Ear Fold
Daith
UB10

Glossary

- **absolute contraindications to massage:** situations in which massage cannot be performed
- **absolute local contraindications for massage:** massage on a certain area must be avoided
- **acupressure:** an Eastern style of massage that presses specific points to change and balance the flow of energy in the body and address specific conditions
- **adductor muscles:** the muscles on the inner thigh near the groin
- **adhesions:** a type of knot in areas where fascia has dried out, fuzzed up, and stuck together. These knots tend to feel sticky, long, and thin, along the fiber of the muscle
- **anemia:** a nutrition condition caused by lack of iron in the blood
- **anterior scalene:** the front muscle in the group of small muscles on the side of the neck
- **arthritis:** worn-down cartilage between two bones resulting in painful bone-on-bone contact
- **atherosclerosis:** plaque buildup in the arteries
- **autoimmune disorder:** when the body attacks its own cells because it cannot recognize them properly
- **Ayurveda:** an ancient system of medicine in India that prescribes daily and seasonal regimens depending on a person's constitution
- **basalt:** lava rock that holds heat well; for use as a hot stone
- **biceps brachii:** the long muscle on the front of the upper arm
- **body mechanics:** the technique of using your body during massage to protect and support the joints and increase the pressure without adding stress to your body
- **bone:** living, growing tissue that provides the framework for the body, with a thick, dense outer layer and a light, spongy inner layer
- **brachial plexus:** bundle of nerves for the arm
- **calcaneal tendon:** the thick tendon at the back of the heel
- **calf muscles:** muscles on the back of the lower leg
- **carpal tunnel:** a tunnel on the palm side of the wrist created by nine tendons and one nerve crossed over by a wide ligament band

- **carpal tunnel syndrome:** nerve condition that occurs in the carpal tunnel when the tendons are thickened or inflamed by overuse or injury, compressing the nerve and causing pain, tingling, numbness, and weakness in the hand and fingers
- **cervical vertebrae:** the seven bones in the neck that guard the spinal cord
- **chronic fatigue syndrome (CFS):** a physical and mental health condition referring to long-term tiredness that is unrelated to the amount of sleep you get
- **complementary and alternative medicine (CAM):** health-care approaches that are not typically part of conventional medical care or that may have origins outside of usual Western practice
- **consent:** permission for something to happen or an agreement to do something
- **cortisol:** the hormone released by the body in response to high levels of stress; in potentially dangerous situations, cortisol raises your heart rate and shuts down less essential systems like digestion, which is important in the body's fight-flight-or-freeze response
- **craniosacral therapy:** a style of massage that tests for the ease and motion of the pulse in the cerebrospinal fluid around the brain and spinal cord
- **Crohn's disease:** inflammation of the lining of the entire digestive tract
- **cumulative trauma disorder (CTD):** wear and tear on the tendons, muscles, and nerves caused by continuous use over an extended period
- **daith:** the point where the ear cartilage sticks out, just above the ear hole
- **deep tissue:** a style of massage using warming strokes and firm pressure to reach deeper layers of muscle and fascia. The person doing the massage uses minimal lotion and incorporates arms and elbows to apply more pressure. It typically focuses on a specific area of muscle pain or tension to release adhesions, break down scar tissue, and realign muscle fibers
- **deltoid ("delts"):** the thick round cap of muscle that covers the top of the shoulder
- **dermatome:** a specific area of the body that one nerve branch from the spine sends messages to. When the nerve is affected anywhere along the dermatome pathway, pain can also happen farther along the pathway
- **diaphragm:** the thick band of muscle that moves up and down to create the inhale and exhale
- **discs:** tissue between the bones of the spine (vertebrae), which prevents friction between them

- **dopamine:** one of the body's pain-relieving hormones that helps with focus
- **edema:** swelling due to fluid pooling in an area of the body
- **effleurage:** a Swedish massage technique used to introduce your touch and warm the muscles that stimulates the nervous system, increases lymph and blood flow, and stretches the tissues; effleurage comes from the French word "effleurer," which means "to skim"
- **electrolytes:** elements essential to muscle function, including sodium, potassium, and magnesium
- **endorphins:** the hormone released by the body that reduces pain and increases feelings of joy
- **energy:** something that flows within the body and affects our consciousness and function; massage therapists in the East and West agree that an energy exchange takes place when we touch another person with intent to heal
- **erector spinae group:** the group of muscles that tuck into both sides of the spine
- **ergonomic:** relating to or designed for efficiency and comfort in the working environment; essential for reducing pain due to poor posture and repetitive motions
- **ethmoid sinus:** empty cavity behind your nose
- **eustachian tube:** the tube that connects the ear to the nose and throat
- **extensor muscles:** muscles on the back of the forearm that move the hand and fingers outward
- **eyestrain:** an eye condition that occurs when our eyes get tired, the muscles of the eye stop working properly, and the surfaces of the eye get too dry
- **fascia:** an interwoven system of connective tissue made of collagen that holds together the entire body by coating your muscles, organs, and nerves and connecting muscles, bones, tendons, ligaments, and blood; when it is healthy, it allows muscle fibers and other tissues to slide, glide, and move freely
- **fatigue:** the feeling of being extremely tired, both physically and mentally, for a prolonged period
- **feathering:** a massage technique that softly stimulates and relaxes the nervous system, much like stroking a cat
- **femur:** upper leg bone
- **fibula:** the smaller lower leg bone

- **flexor muscles:** muscles on the back of the forearm that bend the hand and fingers inward
- **friction:** small, firm movements applied across muscle fibers to separate adhesions, break down scar tissue, and stimulate healing and blood flow, typically used in myofascial release therapy in sports and medical clinics
- **frontal sinus:** empty cavity in the center of your forehead above each eye
- **frontalis:** the muscle on the forehead
- **gastrocnemius:** the surface calf muscle on the back of the lower leg
- **generalized anxiety disorder (GAD):** a common anxiety disorder causing nervousness, irritability, increased heart rate, rapid breathing, fatigue, insomnia, difficulty concentrating, muscle tension, and/or digestive issues
- **gliding:** see effleurage
- **glutes:** the muscles on the buttocks layered on top of each other in the gluteal region
- **gluteus maximus:** the surface gluteal muscle on the buttocks
- **gluteus medius:** the middle gluteal muscle on the buttocks
- **gluteus minimis:** the deepest gluteal muscle on the buttocks
- **gout:** a joint condition where uric acid builds up in the body and deposits crystals in the joints, which cause chronic joint pain and swelling
- **grounding:** a technique of preparing to give or receive a massage by letting go of your own stress and being present in the moment with your partner; allows you to set your intention for your massage, increase your focus, and improve the benefits of the massage for your partner
- **hamstrings:** muscles on the back of the upper leg
- **head:** the rounded end of a bone
- **humerus:** upper arm bone
- **iliacus:** the muscle along the inside of the hipbone
- **iliotibial band (IT band):** the thick band of fascia on the side of the hip and leg
- **inflammatory bowel disease (IBD):** sometimes used to refer to ulcerative colitis and Crohn's disease together
- **infraspinatus:** the muscle on top of the shoulder blade
- **insomnia:** a mental health condition involving difficulty sleeping, whether falling asleep, staying asleep, or waking up in the morning

- **integrative medicine:** an approach to health care that brings conventional and complementary approaches together in a coordinated way; emphasizes a holistic, patient-focused approach to health care and wellness—often including mental, emotional, functional, spiritual, social, and community aspects—and treating the whole person along with well-coordinated care between different providers and institutions
- **intercostal muscles:** the three layers of muscles between each of the ribs
- **irritable bowel syndrome (IBS):** chronic digestive condition
- **ischial tuberosity:** the bony point you feel when you sit on the floor, at the bottom of the glutes where the hamstrings connect
- **joint:** where two or more bones meet
- **kneading:** see petrissage
- **knot:** areas in muscles that feel tight, dense, and sticky; generally three kinds of "knotted" tissue: adhesions, scar tissue, and trigger points
- **lateral epicondylitis:** an inflammatory condition in tendons of the outside edge of the elbow that causes wrist and hand pain
- **latissimus dorsi:** the muscle that covers the mid-back like a wing and attaches to the top of the upper arm
- **levator scapula:** the muscle that runs from the upper corner of the shoulder blade to the neck
- **ligament:** the tissue connecting bone to bone
- **lumbar vertebrae:** 12 bones in the lower spine that guard the spinal cord
- **lymph system:** the waste removal and white blood cell transportation system of the body
- **mandible:** the jaw bone
- **masseter:** the large muscle at the corner where the jaw bone meets the cheek bone and head
- **maxillary sinus:** an empty cavity on either side of your nose below the cheekbones
- **medial epicondylitis:** an inflammatory condition in tendons of the inside edge of the elbow that causes wrist and hand pain
- **middle scalene:** the middle muscle in the group of small muscles on the side of the neck

- **muscle tension:** large areas in muscles that feel tight, dense, and sticky, cause pain, and decrease the range of motion for nearby joints; caused when a muscle contracts and does not release, limiting the flow of blood, oxygen, and nutrients to the area
- **muscle:** the tissue connected to bones that move the skeleton
- **musculoskeletal disorder (MSD):** wear and tear on the tendons, muscles, and nerves caused by continuous use over an extended period
- **nerves:** the body's communication system; uses bundles of long string-like nerve cells called neurons wrapped in fatty cells to rapidly conduct nerve impulses from the brain, spinal cord, skeletal muscles, and other body parts
- **neuron:** long string-like nerve cells that conduct signals from the brain and spinal cord to other parts of the body
- **osteoarthritis:** a joint condition where cartilage on the ends of bones inside the joint wears away due to overuse, leaving the bones exposed to friction and causing rough bony surfaces to develop
- **oxytocin:** a hormone that improves relationship stability
- **patella:** the kneecap
- **pectoralis major ("pecs"):** the muscles on the chest underneath the collarbone
- **pectoralis minor:** the small strap-like muscle that forms the front edge of the armpit
- **pelvis:** the bone in the groin
- **percussion:** see tapotement
- **peroneus group:** the muscles on the side of the lower leg
- **petrissage:** a Swedish massage technique used to compress and release muscles; improves fascia's movement, increases lymph and blood flow, and relaxes muscles; petrissage comes from the French word "pétrir," which means "to knead"
- **piriformis:** the triangle-shaped muscle between the top of the leg bone and the tailbone
- **piriformis syndrome:** a nerve condition that occurs when the sciatic nerve is compressed by muscles in the glutes
- **polyps:** extra tissue in the nose
- **popliteus:** the small muscle on the back of the knee just below the knee crease
- **premenstrual syndrome (PMS):** a combination of physical and emotional symptoms occurring 1 to 2 weeks prior to menstruation due to the change in hormones that create the menstrual cycle

- **pronator teres:** muscle on the forearm that turns the hand palm up or palm down
- **psoas:** a long, slender strip that runs from either side of the spine in the middle back, down through the pelvis, and to the top of the inner thigh bone
- **qi:** the Traditional Chinese Medicine concept of energy that flows in the body along channels (meridians)
- **quadratus lumborum:** a square muscle that attaches to the top of the hip bone (the pelvis), the lower back (lumbar) spine, and the bottom of their ribs
- **quadriceps muscle group ("quads"):** the large group of four muscles on the front of the upper leg
- **rectus femoris:** the big muscle on the front of the thigh that crosses from the upper leg to the hip bone (one of the muscles in the quadriceps group)
- **reflexology:** a style of massage used to relieve tension and treat illness, based on the theory that there are points on the feet, hands, and ears that influence every part of the body
- **Reiki:** a Japanese style of massage that uses energetic work that heals body, mind, and spirit by working with the "subtle vibrational field" that surrounds the human body
- **relative contraindications for massage:** situations where massage may be helpful, but the treatment must be modified in some way to accommodate certain health conditions
- **repetitive motion injury (RMI):** wear and tear on the tendons, muscles, and nerves caused by continuous use over an extended period
- **repetitive strain injury (RSI):** wear and tear on the tendons, muscles, and nerves caused by continuous use over an extended period
- **rheumatoid arthritis:** a typically body-wide inflammation of the fibrous connective tissue around joints
- **rhomboids:** the muscles between the shoulder blade and spine
- **rocking and shaking:** an Eastern massage technique used to sedate the nervous system, much like rocking a crying baby or sitting in a rocking chair; it is also used in Western massage sessions as a warming tool to evaluate an area's movement and tension, and as a sports massage technique to release the muscles before and after an athletic event
- **rotator cuff:** a group of four muscles, including supraspinatus, infraspinatus, teres minor, and subscapularis, which keep the end (or head) of the upper arm bone (the humerus) in its socket

- **sacrum:** five fused bones in the lowest part of the spine
- **sartorius:** the long strap-like muscle that runs from the outer edge of the hip bone down the front of the leg to the inner knee
- **scalenes:** the small muscles on the side of the neck
- **scar tissue:** a type of knot in previously injured areas where thick white fibers were quickly laid down in all directions to repair gaps in tissue; these knots tend to feel harder and less movable than others
- **sciatic nerve:** the thick nerve running from the lumbar spine through the gluteal region and down the leg
- **sciatica:** irritation of the sciatic nerve running through the glutes and down the leg
- **secret knot:** see serratus posterior superior
- **serotonin:** one of the hormones released by the body that helps with pain relief, irritability and cravings; also an essential hormone for melatonin production, which regulates awake and sleep cycles
- **serratus posterior superior:** the muscles on the ribs underneath the shoulder blade; known as the "secret knot" because it is usually missed in massages for shoulder tension, since it lives under the shoulder blade and cannot be massaged unless the shoulder blade is moved out of the way by bringing the arm overhead
- **Shiatsu:** a Japanese acupressure style of massage that uses finger pressure to move the body's energy along meridians to restore balance and health
- **soleus:** the deep calf muscle on the back of the lower leg, particularly a few inches above the inner ankle
- **sphenoid sinus:** an empty cavity behind your nose
- **spinal cord:** nerve tissue inside the spine
- **spinal stenosis:** narrowing of the spinal cord canal
- **sports massage:** a style of massage intended to help athletes before and after events
- **stacked fingers:** holding two or more fingers together with arched fingers to support and protect the joints of the fingers and hand during massage
- **stacked hands:** holding the hands together with arched fingers to support and protect the joints of the fingers and hand during massage
- **sternocleidomastoid:** the big muscle on the front of the neck

- **stress:** any situation that requires a response from the body or brain; a natural part of life
- **stretching:** an Eastern and Western technique used in Thai, Shiatsu, sports, and medical massage to remind the muscle how long it can be and help retain that length
- **subclavius:** the small muscle under the collarbone and above the first rib
- **suboccipitals:** the muscles at the base of the head
- **subscapularis:** the muscle tucking inside the front of the shoulder blade
- **supported thumb:** a hand position for massage holding the thumb against the fingers or between the first and second knuckle to support and protect the joints of the thumb
- **supraspinatus:** the muscle on top of the shoulder blade
- **Swedish massage:** modern massage techniques, including gliding (effleurage), kneading (petrissage), friction, vibration, and tapping (tapotement)
- **tapotement:** a Swedish massage technique used to stimulate the nervous system and lymph and blood flow; tapotement comes from the French word "tapoter," which means to tap or drum
- **tapping:** see tapotement
- **temporal bone:** the bone at the side of the head
- **temporalis:** the muscle on the side of the head above the ears
- **temporomandibular joint syndrome (TMJ syndrome):** chronic tension in the jaw causing jaw pain, clicking, ear pain and ringing, dizziness, tension headaches, and toothaches
- **tendinitis:** tendon inflammation
- **tendinopathy:** tendon pain
- **tendons:** tissue that connects muscle to bone
- **tensor fascia latae:** the small thumb-sized muscle on the outer upper leg
- **teres minor:** the muscle on the outside edge of the shoulder blade that attaches to the upper arm bone
- **Thai massage:** a style of massage from Thailand that uses waves of gentle pressure and yoga-like stretching to gradually stretch the entire body and move energy along channels
- **third eye:** the point between your partner's eyebrows and just above bridge of their nose
- **thoracic outlet syndrome:** a nerve condition when the nerves that run from the neck to the arm are compressed in one or more outlets between muscles and bone
- **thoracic vertebrae:** 12 bones in the upper spine that guard the spinal cord

- **tibia:** shin bone on the front of the lower leg
- **tibialis anterior:** shin muscle on the front of the lower leg
- **Traditional Chinese Medicine:** an approach to health care that believes the body's energy, or qi, flows along established meridians, and dysfunction occurs when qi is stagnant or overabundant
- **trapezius ("traps"):** the muscle that covers the back in a diamond shape from the base of the head out to the shoulders and down to the spine at the middle of the back
- **triceps brachii:** the long muscle on the back of the upper arm
- **trigger finger:** a stiff tendon that causes your finger to catch when it is straightened
- **trigger point:** a type of knot in areas where muscle contraction has cut off the flow of blood and nutrients to the area, resulting in microscopic contractions that don't let go; known as a "hyper-irritable spot in a taut band of muscle" that refers pain to other areas in the body when pressed
- **trigger point therapy:** a style of massage used in medical massage to address trigger points, which cause pain, complicate pain, and mimic pain. It uses direct, focused pressure on these hyper-irritable spots in taut bands of muscle to release them and restore blood flow, functions and strength to the muscle
- **Tui Na:** a Chinese acupressure style of massage that uses rhythmic compressions and acupressure to massage soft tissue and improve energy flow
- **ulcerative colitis:** inflammation of the lining of the colon
- **vastus lateralis:** the thick muscle above the outside of the knee (a muscle in the quadriceps group)
- **vibration:** a massage technique that lightly shakes an area of the recipient's body, using vibrations produced in by the massaging hands and arms; can soothe irritated nerves, increase blood and lymph flow, and relax the muscles

Resources

Acupuncture.com: Gateway to Chinese Medicine, Health, and Wellness
Great resource for information on Traditional Chinese Medicine, meridians, and acupressure points.

American Chronic Pain Association (ACPA): TheACPA.org
Research and information on dealing with chronic pain.

American Headache Society: AmericanHeadacheSociety.org
Research and information on dealing with headaches.

American Massage Therapy Association: AMTAmassage.org
Research and information on the benefits of massage therapy.

Anxiety and Depression Association of America: ADAA.org
Research and information on dealing with anxiety and depression.

Arthritis Foundation: Arthritis.org
Research and information on dealing with arthritis.

Biel, Andrew. *Trail Guide to the Body: How to Locate Muscles, Bones, and More*, 6th ed. Books of Discovery, 2019.
Excellent resource for learning about the muscles and other structures of the musculoskeletal system.

Centers for Disease Control: CDC.gov
National organization for research and information on dealing with chronic and acute conditions.

Cleveland Clinic: My.ClevelandClinic.org/health
Detailed and trustworthy resource for all health issues and questions.

Davies, Clair, and Amber Davies. *The Trigger Point Therapy Workbook: Your Self-Treatment Guide for Pain Relief*, **3rd ed. Oakland, CA: New Harbinger Publications, 2013.**
Fantastic resource that explains trigger points in layman's terms and teaches you how to massage them yourself.

Donnelly, Joseph M. et al. *Travell, Simons and Simons' Myofascial Pain and Dysfunction: The Trigger Point Manual*, **3rd ed. Philadelphia, PA: Wolters Kluwer, 2018.**
The original resource and research for trigger point therapy, updated.

doTERRA.com
Great resource for information on the uses and benefits of essential oils, and for purchasing high-quality oils as well.

Georgetown University's Center on an Aging Society: HPI.Georgetown.edu/archive/agingsociety/profiles
Great resource for research and recommendations on musculoskeletal pain.

Healthline.com
Great, simple resource for any and things massage and acupressure (as well as other health conditions).

Mayo Clinic: MayoClinic.org
Detailed and trustworthy resource for all health issues and questions.

Migraine Research Foundation: MigraineResearchFoundation.org
Research and information on dealing with migraines.

National Center for Complementary and Integrative Health: NCCIH.NIH.gov/health/massage
National website for health research and information on massage and other alternative therapies.

National Headache Foundation: Headaches.org
Research and information on dealing with headaches.

National Institutes for Health, U.S. National Library for Medicine: MedlinePlus.gov
National website for health research and information.

Salvo, Susan. *Mosby's Pathology for Massage Therapists, 4th ed.* St. Louis, MO: Elsevier, 2017.
Excellent resource for looking up ailments and getting a simple explanation of the resource and how to use massage to help.

PainScience.com
Great, detailed website with good advice for aches, pains, and injuries. Explains trigger points, myofascial pain syndromes, the nature of pain, and lots more, including specific recommendations for massage for many kinds of issues.

Young Living Essential Oils: YoungLiving.com
Great resource for information on the uses and benefits of essential oils.

References

Anxiety and Depression Association of America. "Understanding GAD—and the Symptoms." Accessed January 13, 2020. ADAA.org/understanding-anxiety/generalized-anxiety-disorder-gad.

Dahlhamer, J., J. Lucas, C. Zelaya, R. Nahin, S. Mackey, L. DeBar, R. Kerns, M. Von Korff, L. Porter, and C. Helmick. "Prevalence of Chronic Pain and High-Impact Chronic Pain Among Adults—United States, 2016." *Morbidity and Mortality Weekly Report*. 67, no. 36 (September 14, 2018):1001–06. doi: 10.15585/mmwr.mm6736a2.

Field, T., M. Hernandez-Reif, M. Diego, S. Schanberg, and C. Kuhn. "Cortisol Decreases and Serotonin and Dopamine Increase following Massage Therapy." *International Journal of Neuroscience*. 115, no. 10 (October 2005): 1397–413. doi: 10.1080/00207450590956459.

Field, Tiffany. "Massage Therapy Research Review." *Complementary Therapies in Clinical Practice*. 20, no. 4 (November 2014): 224–29. doi: 10.1016/j.ctcp.2014.07.002.

Georgetown University. "Chronic Back Pain." Accessed February 11, 2020. HPI.Georgetown.edu/backpain.

Heart of Wellness. "Eustachian Tube Massage." Published March 6, 2017. HeartOfWellness.org/eustachian-tube-massage.

United States Bone and Joint Initiative. "Low Back Pain." Accessed February 11, 2020. BoneAndJointBurden.org/fourth-edition/iiaa0/low-back-pain.

Mayo Clinic. "Massage: Get in Touch with Its Many Benefits." Published. October 6, 2018. MayoClinic.org/healthy-lifestyle/stress-management/in-depth/massage/art-20045743.

National Institutes of Health: National Center for Complementary and Integrative Health. "Complementary, Alternative, or Integrative Health: What's In a Name?" Last modified July 2018. NCCIH.NIH.gov/health/complementary-alternative-or-integrative-health-whats-in -a-name.

National Institutes of Health: National Center for Complementary and Integrative Health. "Massage Therapy: What You Need To Know." Last modified May 2019. NCCIH.NIH.gov /health/massage-therapy-what-you-need-to-know.

Natural Eye Care. "CVS: Computer Eye Strain." Accessed February 11, 2020. NaturalEyeCare .com/eye-conditions/computer-eye-strain.

Ramachandran, V. S., and S. Blakeslee. *Phantoms in the Brain: Probing the Mysteries of the Human Mind.* New York: William Morrow, 1999.

The Ayurveda Experience. "Abhyanga: Ayurvedic Massage Benefits." May 18, 2017. Accessed September 2, 2019. Products.TheAyurvedaExperience.com/blogs/tae /abhyanga-ayurvedic-massage-benefits.

The International Center for Reiki Training. "What Is the History of Reiki?" Accessed September 2, 2019. Reiki.org/faqs/what-history-reiki#usui.

Upledger Institute International. "CST [Craniosacral Therapy] FAQs." Accessed September 2, 2019. Upledger.com/therapies/faq.php.

Vibe-Fersum, K., P. O'Sullivan, J. Skouen, A. Smith, A. Kvåle. "Efficacy of Classification-based Cognitive Functional Therapy in Patients with Non-specific Chronic Low Back Pain: A Randomized Controlled Trial." *European Journal of Pain.* 17, no. 6 (July 2013): 916–28. doi: 10.1002/j.1532-2149.2012.00252.x.

Index

About the Author

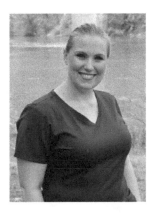 **Jennifer Love** is a massage therapy instructor at the Sacramento campus of National Holistic Institute, a college of massage therapy. She also runs her medical massage clinic, Integrative Massage Therapy, in midtown Sacramento, where she collaborates with doctors, chiropractors, physical therapists, and other health-care professionals to provide neuromuscular massage therapy and health education to patients dealing with chronic pain and muscle tension. Jennifer is passionate about the movement to integrate massage therapy into the health-care industry.

Jennifer is married to Calith Sprock. They have three boys, Jefferson, Jackson, and Joshua—and another one is on the way! They love Jesus, board games, cooking together, and camping in the great outdoors (especially traveling to national parks and Cub Scouting). Jennifer loves to coach her boys in soccer and baseball. She is also a worship leader and kids' pastor at Jesus Culture Sacramento, a charismatic church in Folsom, California.